Pocket A-Z of
Natural Healthcare

GW00496545

Other books by Belinda Grant Viagas

The Detox Diet Book

Natural Remedies for Common Complaints

Natural Healthcare for Women

Pocket A-Z of Natural Healthcare

BELINDA GRANT VIAGAS

NEWLEAF

Newleaf
an imprint of Gill & Macmillan Ltd
Goldenbridge
Dublin 8
with associated companies throughout the world

0 7522 2126 4

This is a revised, updated and expanded edition
of *Alternative Health: A–Z of Natural Healthcare*
by Belinda Grant published in 1993 by Optima.

Print origination by SX Composing DTP, Rayleigh, Essex
Printed by The Guernsey Press

A catalogue record is available for this book
from the British Library.

1 3 5 4 2

DEDICATION

To Nora Viagas, my mother and friend, with love

ADVICE TO THE READER

ACKNOWLEDGEMENTS

Kathryn Scott's skilful computer teaching was a welcome gift, and I treasure the richness of our friendship. Gordon Scott Wise, Senior Editor at Boxtree/Macmillan encouraged this book to shine, with his brilliant eye for detail and clear overview, and I am glad of his patience. 'Pearl' opened many windows for me. I would especially like to thank Maureen and Rob Lloyd-Owen of Poise Stress Management Consultancy for their work on NLP and for their loving friendship, and Mark Reidy from Neal's Yard Therapy Rooms for his work on Tongue Diagnosis and in sharing his knowledge of oriental medicine. The original chapter on healing was written as a result of interviews with Betty Balcombe who gave generously of her time. Simon Tapsell was a very welcome Fnord bringer, and Sandra Boyes was instrumental in getting the first version ready for publication.

CONTENTS

INTRODUCTION

This book is about the wide-ranging, comprehensive system of healthcare that is naturopathy. It is supportive, life-enhancing, effective, safe, and often simple.

The healthcare umbrella embraces a range of different therapies, which are listed in alphabetical order. Each entry contains information on natural forms of healthcare, methods of treatment and practices, what you can expect the therapy to do for you, and how best to use this form of treatment for yourself at home. It is a reference for self-help and information, and many chapters include practical advice for managing and treating minor ailments. The therapy sections also outline what each particular specialty has to offer, and what you can expect from a visit to a practitioner.

Alternative medicine is a huge subject, containing many different philosophies and ways for approaching individual health and a variety of practical applications. This book is about natural healthcare and contains information on all those therapies which support the body's natural function – its self-regulating mechanisms – and you can use most of these yourself at home.

The rich abundance of therapies and natural healthcare

methods makes our need for information greater than ever, and it is every bit as important to be able to make informed choices about our healthcare as it is in every other area of our lives. Those of us who have consulted a practitioner may want to know more about how and why their treatments work. Trying it out for yourself is a very good way to see how compatible a particular branch of natural healthcare is, and many therapies can be sampled at home before making the decision to pursue a particular one with a practitioner.

This holistic form of healing is all about recognising the strength of the connections between body, mind and spirit. An understanding of the integrity of our experience is a springboard to good health. When we can discover the root cause of any disease or disharmony, then we know where to look for healing.

This book is a comprehensive guide to the many natural options available to us. Under their own umbrella of Naturopathy, a wide variety of approaches and skills are to be found. Not least among the reasons for such choice is one of the primary objectives of this philosophy – that the work is not so much in curing a patient, but in educating each person to live in harmony with their own unique recipe for full health.

NATURAL HEALTHCARE

Natural healthcare provides us with a myriad of different ways of restoring health and balance to all levels of our being. Its three main 'arms' or areas of concern are with the person's physical structure (see Osteopathy and Chiropractic, Kinesiology, Bodywork, Massage, etc), how the body works, (see Nutrition, Herbs, Juicing, etc) and the links between the body and the psycho-emotional and the spiritual self (see Body Forms, Counselling, Healing, etc.).

Many of these healing techniques have been known to us for centuries. Eating herbs with a meal for their medicinal properties stemmed from learning the therapeutic values of all locally grown foods. From the time our ancestors were hunter-gatherers, we have known the importance of remaining physically active, and of moderating and varying our food intake. And, as social creatures, we have always known the value of sharing our thoughts, ideas and feelings with others.

Some of the therapies and practices included here have evolved more recently. Neuro-linguistic Programming (NLP) and Cranio-sacral therapy, for example, embrace very new-age concepts of holism and effectiveness, yet their roots are firmly planted in the history of healing. As practitioners and patients bring their own individual skills together, and as we continue to push back the limits of our understanding about the magnificence and variety of our human experience, so new therapies are born.

In recent years, we in the West have embraced a particular form of medicine and made it mainstream. Allopathic medicine is now accepted as the norm – the GP or MD whom we visit practises it, and it is what all our hospitals provide. We have come to know it as medicine, yet it is only one branch of our vast tree of knowledge concerning health.

With our growing awareness of ourselves as multi-dimensional beings with emotional, spiritual, physical and social needs, we realize how these distinct areas of our lives all overlap and influence one another. All the therapies in this book share a view of the individual as comprising more than just a physical body, and the belief that the integrity of *all* parts of a person is central to their health.

We, each of us, have our own unique recipe for full health that is quite unlike that of anybody else's – in just the same way that we look different, sound different, and have different personalities. The idea that full health involves emotional and spiritual as well as physical well-being is by no means new. Hippocrates spoke at length about the integrity of the individual and the importance of assessing and understanding the person as a whole being rather than concentrating only on the disease. In taking the Hippocratic oath, allopathic medics have taken only part of a truth and used it out of context; taken an active principle and disregarded the rest.

4

Of course, not all natural therapies offer a comprehensive approach, but with few exceptions they recognize the existence and importance of an holistic overview. Simple, life-supporting techniques have no side effects, and most are complementary in the widest sense – they not only enhance the health of the individual but can work effectively alongside one another. Combining the use of aromatherapy oils with flower remedies and herbs, for example, would be safe, effective and pleasant.

All naturopathic therapies seek to strengthen and support the individual's own life force or vitality. Through harnessing the elements of nature and developing ways of working with them, we uncover a complete system of medicine that is safe, effective and completely accessible – we can all use it every day if we need to. It is all about educating ourselves about our own needs, and deepening our relationship with ourselves and with the natural world – our world. The use of diet, herbs, water, physical contact, etc., forms a natural method of primary healthcare, providing everyday solutions to everyday difficulties.

Naturopathy also looks to the maintenance of full health and, as such, includes a number of methods which are aimed specifically at strengthening the individual and reinforcing their ability to remain disease-free. It also forms an important preventive and life-enhancing function by searching out and addressing the underlying causes of an imbalance, rather than focusing on the presenting symptoms.

We cannot be healthy in isolation; the effects of the environment, pollutants, and food additives such as preservatives, colourings, flavourings, emulsifiers, bleaches and stabilizers all influence the way in which we function. We are what we eat; this is how our healing functions are fuelled, and growth and vitality depend upon regular fuel. When the energy we provide is substandard or adulterated, it does not enable us to live well.

The continual need to fight airborne pollutants and other allergens can lead to our immune system being over-taxed. The presence in a diet of a wide range of toxins can soon lead to poor digestion and assimilation of nutrients, and great internal biochemical confusion. Such physiological stress can lead in turn to faulty elimination and a lack of tone and vitality in the tissues and cells. It's like running a fantastic new performance engine on low-grade diesel. It is at this stage that we may begin to manifest 'sub-clinical' feelings of tiredness – feeling below par, a general malaise, lowered resistance to viruses, bacteria and infection, and begin to run ourselves down physically, emotionally and mentally. We are not, as a rule, given enough information about the foods we eat – labelling is less than helpful, most of our fresh fruits and vegetables are chemically grown and treated with a cocktail of synthetic products, and now we are seeing more and more foods that have been irradiated and genetically changed.

We also need to know more about how our bodies work. Although we all have individual differences, the majority of our 'workings' are the same, and a fundamental aspect of living well is in knowing how to. It is easier to make decisions about our immediate environment, our diet, even our social habits, when we understand our real needs and are informed as to how to meet them. How many of us would choose, for instance, to deprive ourselves of sunshine? Yet we often attribute a low priority in our busy schedules to time spent outdoors. And where, on that long list, comes the development of personal skills such as self-awareness and analysis?

It is often left to the individual, in their search for personal growth, to discover a spiritual aspect to their lives; to understand their own psychology and, particularly in our society, to learn and value the importance of self-nourishment.

Our own basic vitality is called many different things throughout the world. It is Chi (China), Ki or Qi (Pacific rim), Prana or Manna (Asia) or spirit. It is the universal spark, the energy of life. As living, evolving organisms we are always looking towards full health and the more ways we can find to enhance and facilitate this move, the better. In our quest for the best, the optimum health, ease of function, happiness and well-being, it is not intervention but support that is needed.

By listening to our own needs, and by learning to interpret them, we can begin to encourage our momentum towards full health. When a symptom of ill health manifests itself, we can choose to ignore it, or to see it as a sign which is pointing the way towards an area in need of our attention. We can liken the body (our physical home) to a house (our material home). On discovering a crack in one of the walls, we would have a number of options – to cover it with a coat of paint for example; or to investigate and see whether there might be some subsidence, or shaky foundations.

The choice may well be governed by our sense of responsibility. In our own home, such a crack may lead us to pursue many avenues to ascertain whether there were, indeed, any structural problems; or if it was a simple case of bad decorating or plastering. Alternatively, we might just phone the landlords and let them know about it, or hang a picture over it and do nothing. This analogy reflects so well the attitudes that many of us have towards our own health, and highlights our options – we can embody our lives, or see it as somebody else's responsibility.

A mainstay of the nature-cure philosophy is that health is an individual process and an individual responsibility. The life force is not a conscious will that can be determined, or an unconscious drive that is open to our understanding. It exists as a spirit or source of energy, and to intervene in its process is a tremendous responsibility. Any intervention requires careful management, and even raises a moral question.

Surgery can be seen as the ultimate in interventionist treatment – vital and life-saving on occasion, but an invasive assault on the body. Medication is somewhat more insidious, because many chemicals and pharmaceutical drugs interfere with the body's own necessary functions. Pain-killers, for example, do nothing to relieve the condition, they just block our awareness of the pain, and generate an enormous amount of physical work in expelling the by-products from our system afterwards. In an emergency they may be considered, but for regular use they are surely too hazardous. Besides, this has always seemed to me a bit like hearing a baby cry and responding by going out to buy a pair of earplugs. Or moving into a home with an elegant and sophisticated alarm system – the latest, up-to-the-minute technological whiz, and working hard to disconnect it as soon as one of the bells sounds.

Intervention, then, may be seen as a serious move – warranted on occasion but needing to be treated with respect, and placed in its proper perspective as an emergency decision, not a routine choice. It is rarely an answer rather than a response, and there is usually an easier, simpler way. Some alternative therapies can also be seen as invasive or interventionist – those that routinely puncture or burn the skin; or that override the person's own conscious process. This book adheres to the holistic philosophy of nature cure, and explores only those therapies that do not violate the integrity of the individual.

There are other systems of healthcare: Kahuna healing, Ayurvedic medicine and Shamanism, for example; naturopathy does not have the answers for everybody, but it can do a lot! In its simplicity it is deeply impressive; not just in its efficacy, but also in the ease with which it can be used by so many people.

How to Use This Book

Each alphabetical entry defines a natural therapy or practice. Often the information from one chapter overlaps with others; Herbs, for example, have their own entry and are also included as a useful aid within Hydrotherapy, and the essential oils are discussed separately as Aromatherapy.

Whether the therapies involve visits to a practitioner or are designed for more individual use, many of the chapters include suggestions and advice for home use. There are first-aid tips and reference tables to assist with a range of minor complaints. Obviously, these cannot replace individual advice from your natural healthcare or other practitioner.

Many of the suggestions in this book are not about any specific therapy but are a part of living life in good health. Our need for quiet, outdoor contact and the company of others, for example, can often be as essential to our own well-being as more defined health measures.

Each chapter includes a resource section with suggestions for further reading and contacts.

Finding a Practitioner

A naturopath or natural healthcare practitioner will have knowledge or experience of all of the therapies contained in this book. Their job is very much like that of a natural GP – providing a diagnosis, and treating or referring patients on to a specialist in a particular field. They fulfil a role as primary care provider, and can supply an ongoing focus when different therapies are being used. Healthcare is becoming more specialized, and new forms or techniques emerge regularly. This can only add to our rich repertoire of healing resources. As individual therapies become more defined there is a greater than ever need to develop an overview.

When I began in practice, there were few aromatherapists; it was mostly used by massage therapists, rather than being a specialization in its own right. There were no practitioners who worked solely with Flower Remedies, or with muscle testing techniques (applied kinesiology) and lymphatic massage was one of the treatments used by naturopaths. Now these are all specific therapies, with their own practitioners. The world of natural healthcare is growing and developing as more practitioners unite their own unique personal attributes, and synthesize techniques and approaches.

11

It is important to know what you are looking for when choosing a practitioner, and the main distinction is between those who can act as a primary care provider, and those who are specialists in their own, less broad, field of expertise. Your naturopath or natural healthcare practitioner will be able to provide you with referrals to other practitioners for specialist care. Their treatments will cover three main 'arms' of healthcare – some form of bodywork, so that the physical and structural problems can be addressed; a type of counselling; and some form of nutritional work. Individual practitioners may specialize in herbs, for instance, or supplements and this is one of the things you can find out during your initial research.

The world of alternative medicine is currently undergoing a process of change. The profession's associations and training colleges are coming together to find where they may standardize their approaches, and work in greater harmony with each other. This is leading to the formation of new qualifications and methods of recognition as colleges merge their curricula and change their titles. It is also creating a large body of professionals who may at any one time be unaligned or between classifications. Finding a practitioner, therefore, has not been made any easier in the short term, although this will change as the colleges and professional bodies for each discipline become able to provide a list of practitioners who have attended or completed their courses together with details on the curriculum and information leaflets.

Choosing a practitioner must always be a matter of personal concern – most professional registers are filled by those who have completed a course of training, but that is not the only factor that should govern your choice. Not all practitioners join their relevant associations upon qualifying, and experienced therapists may let their membership lapse.

Any areas of expertise or speciality, experience, and the rapport you establish with the practitioner are all important. By far the best way to find a practitioner is through some form of personal recommendation (ask your friends, pharmacist, GP, healthfood shop manager), but where this is not possible, use the registers as a starting point, and interview the practitioner in an initial 'phone call or short appointment. Your health and your body are among your greatest assets. It is worth taking time to find the right person who will be sympathetic to your needs and be able to provide you with professional care and advice.

AFFIRMATIONS

These techniques for encouraging change and affirming or enlivening a vision may be verbal, mental or written. They are a powerful tool for change and can be employed just about anywhere and at any time. They are a strong self-help measure that will reinforce your intentions, and can also be used to support and enhance any system of healthcare or specific health measures.

Affirmations can take many forms. Simply, they are an aid to establishing new ways of being, or focusing the individual on a specific thing. 'Every day in every way I am getting better' is a classic example, albeit a rather global one. Affirmations or 'Positive Thought Repetitions' (PTRs) are often most effective when extremely specific and personal, and it helps if they are time-related too, e.g. 'Today's the day I ...', or 'Now is the time for ...'.

These sayings can be thought aloud, written down, or focused on and repeated silently. Twenty-five seems to be a magic number for repetitions, and many people use beads or knots in a piece of string to count them out, although fingers will do just as well. It is thought that these may be the root of Christians counting out their prayers on rosary beads, and of the Greek tradition of worry beads.

Speaking affirmations out loud harnesses a lot of energy – in much the same way as prayers, incantations and mantras call on the energy of all the times they have been spoken in the past.

Like most other ways of achieving change, the effectiveness of these PTRs seems to depend on the energy and commitment with which they are used. I have known people work with affirmations for an assortment of things from finding or selling houses to improving skin conditions – all with great success.

The metre or rhythm of each affirmation is important, so a simple, tuneful and specific saying works best – 'Today's the day I begin to recover' or 'Now I'm starting to make myself better' rather than: 'I am ready to start to improve the condition of my health.' If the affirmation can rhyme, so much the better – this is a short-cut to activating the subconscious, or quiet self, which can do so much towards enabling you to achieve your vision. Good examples are: 'Now's the time my ..... is fine', and 'Now it's revealed, my ..... is healed'.

Visualizing the completed wish is a powerful aid that works very well alongside affirmations. The more ways you can find to work towards enabling something to occur, the more techniques to focus you on your desire, and the more time spent imaging it as reality, the more likely it is to occur.

Affirmations are a good way of formalizing the tickertape, or unspoken thoughts, which are always flowing through our heads. This background noise of criticism, praise, or general chit-chat is ignored by us most of the time – we regard it rather like an old familiar friend whose story is known by us only too well. Whether this voice is a pessimistic, blaming conscience/devil, or a rich, rewarding, encouraging angel, its energy can be harnessed and used to focus consciously on what we need in our lives. Imagine if all that muttering were to be transformed into clear words of active encouragement, confirming what we seek to make true about ourselves and our lives. This is the real power of affirmations.

Affirmations can be used whenever you have a spare moment during the day, although it is a good idea to set aside a specific time as well. Spending ten minutes at the beginning and end of each day on a variety of techniques that will make your vision a reality is a good habit to get into. Beyond that, any time you may make will reaffirm your commitment to achieving your goal. Many psychics, counsellors and therapists will help clients devise their own affirmations as a positive way of continuing the work done in the session, and to encourage reliance on the individual's own unique power to make happen the life that they choose.

Creating Successful Affirmations

- listen to your heart, clear your motivation, and be sure about what you want
- be precise and as specific as possible
- relate your affirmation to the time and space you are now in
- find a tuneful, rhythmic way for the words to flow
- look for a way to make the affirmation rhyme

- attach as much energy as possible by reinforcing your affirmation with visualizations and spending time on repetitions
- repeat your affirmation in blocks of 25, as often as you choose
- be prepared to experience the change you are working for.

Further Reading

Piero Ferucci, *What We May Be*, Crucible Thorsons Publishing
Kenneth Meadows, *The Medicine Way*, Element Books
Barbara Sher with Annie Gottlieb, *Wishcraft*, Ballantine

ALEXANDER TECHNIQUE

This is a system of physical realignment in which the emphasis is on re-educating the body's postural muscles (see also Feldenkrais Method, p 98). The technique works with the conscious holding patterns that occur in muscles, and seeks to rebalance the whole body. If the postural muscles are working at an optimum, then ease of movement will naturally follow. The client or student is encouraged to relearn ways of moving and holding themselves, so that they can move and work more effectively and easily. The new way of moving, or performing a task is repeated until the new habit is learned.

The 'correct' or most relaxed position is one which allows you to move with the most ease, and so simple movements are repeated until the body learns to do them in a relaxed way. This usually involves the teacher or practitioner exerting some restraining or supporting pressure on the body to maintain it in the right position.

The Alexander Technique is popular with actors, musicians and others who use their body as a means of expression, or who do physical work. It originated in Australia where an actor, F.M. Alexander, looked to his body to see exactly what it was that he was doing that was causing him difficulties with his voice production. Over years of study he observed the postural changes in his body – the tense and habitual poses that he struck – and learned how not to do them. He observed that healthy children below the age of about three years move in a perfectly balanced and co-ordinated way, but as they grow older, they start to manifest less beneficial body habits. These are learned through imitating parents, integrating emotions physically, and through faulty experience and poor education. The essence of the Alexander Technique is refreshing the body and renewing that childlike ease of movement through conscious control.

On your first visit to an Alexander teacher you may be surprised to find few props other than a chair, a couch, and a few mirrors. One of the first exercises you will learn is how to stand up and sit down correctly, without causing strain or discomfort. Most of us get up from a seat by leaning forwards and leading with our head. In an Alexander session you will begin learning how to position yourself with your feet underneath you, so that your legs can take the strain of your weight, working to raise and lower you without your head having much to do with the motion. The teacher may gently hold your head, or place a hand on your back between your shoulder blades in order to make sure that your back remains straight, and your head stays in one place. It feels very strange at first, but with practice it is quite easy to feel when you are doing it the right way.

A relaxed posture is really important. It not only ensures ease of movement, but goes a long way towards preventing some of the structural problems so common in older age. Good posture means that there will be good tone in the diaphragm which will improve breathing (and voice production), and assist with all your abdominal functions. Ease of movement means that the body is moving in the way it was designed, without causing any strain or discomfort, or excessive wear and tear on any of the joints. This all makes it easier to feel relaxed and comfortable in your body.

Each visit to an Alexander teacher will last between thirty minutes to one hour. A full course of treatments is necessary to learn new postural habits for the whole body, and, of course, there is much practising to be done between appointments. The number of treatments will depend on the individual, but around thirty would be an average.

Alexander teachers will often work alongside osteopaths or chiropractors who will be able to correct any structural problems before, or early into, a course of treatments. Obviously, these two therapies complement each other enormously – postural retraining cannot be successful in the presence of spinal misalignment, and there is little benefit in correcting bony displacements without re-educating the individual how to use their body well.

It is quite common to feel remarkably changed and physically lighter during or after an Alexander session, and most people recognize that they are moving much more easily, although occasional aches and pains appear while the new postures are being learned.

If you have a keen eye, you may well be able to spot someone who has taken a course of Alexander Technique at quite a distance – the way in which they move, and a certain quality to their stance marks them out among others who do not feel so comfortable in their bodies.

If you stand up straight and imagine yourself suspended from your sternum, or chest bone, you will immediately experience a release of tension in your neck and shoulders. Your chin should be able to settle back a little, and your head is then delicately balanced on the top of your neck. This will give you a taste of the physical changes that can occur when your body structure is working at its best.

Stand quite still, and imagine a wire suspended from the heavens, which is delicately attached along the length of your chest bone. Feel as the wire is held firmly, how your sternum lifts, taking your whole rib cage along with it. Notice how your posture shifts – your weight may settle back into your heels, and your arms will feel freer as your whole shoulder and neck area open up and are less congested. Your neck will also feel as though it is lengthening, and any tension in your jaw should begin to release.

Perfect rest position

Alexander teachers suggest a position that allows the whole body to be perfectly relaxed, therefore benefiting the mind and the whole person. Lie on your back on a flat surface (the floor, or a bed will be fine) where you can be comfortable and undisturbed. Place a small flat pillow or a soft book underneath your head. Keep your legs out straight, and bend your arms at the elbow so that your hands come in and rest loosely on your abdomen. Relax your hands and feet, and take a few full, easy breaths. Remain in this position for five to ten minutes each day to revitalize the body and refresh the mind.

Finding out More
The Professional Association of Alexander Teachers
Madian
Iorwerth Avenue
Aberystwyth
Dyfed SY23 1EW
Tel: 01970 617586
Society of Teachers of the Alexander Technique
10 London House
266 Fulham Road
London SW10 9EL
Tel: 0171 351 0828

Further Reading

F.M. Alexander, *The Use of Self*, E.P. Dutton, New York
Glen Park, *The Art of Changing*, Ashgrove Press
Chris Stevens, *Alexander Technique*, Optima.

AROMATHERAPY

This is any treatment using the aromatic or essential oils obtained from a variety of plants for their medicinal properties.

These essential oils are extracted from the leaves, stems, roots, or any part of the plant in a variety of ways; using water extraction, heat treatment, or oil basing. Once extracted, the oils can be used in their pure and extremely potent form, or diluted using a carrier oil.

The pure oils can be taken internally in drop form, and used to treat a variety of health concerns – it is important that only the purest oils are used in this way, and they should never be taken without the advice and monitoring of a qualified and experienced practitioner. This method of treatment is used throughout Europe, and is gaining popularity in the UK.

The most common way of using the oils is in dilute form, in a base or carrier oil. These can then be added to bath water, or further diluted in oil and used in aromatherapy massage.

The essential properties of the plant oils impart different qualities – some sedating, like basil, others stimulating, like rosemary, or balancing, like geranium. There are essential oils that will affect a number of physical and emotional responses, e.g. calm the nerves, stimulate digestion and help depression. The aroma of the oil is one of its most active properties. Smell is the quickest route to the brain, and the smell association area of the brain is right next to the part concerned with memory. This explains the evocative nature of aromas – how they can conjure up memories and feelings from times long gone. This also accounts for many of the mood–changing qualities of aromatherapy treatments.

Aromatherapists will usually use a light massage as their way of covering you with the oils. Almost all of the oils can be used safely in this way at home. The pure oils should never be applied directly to the skin, because they can burn.

The oil can be added to bath water, as a therapeutic addition to a foot bath, for self-massage, steam inhalations, and either dispersed in water or burnt as a room scent. The powerful effect of these oils should not be underestimated, and as a general rule, add just three drops to a teaspoon of carrier oil for scenting the bath, and five drops to a saucer full of carrier oil for massage.

When adding essential oils to the bath, make sure that the door remains closed, and that the aroma and the steam remain in the room for you to inhale as you soak. You can buy bath oils which contain essential oils in their dilute form, so check the label to see how much you need to add.

Special oil burners can be used to scent a room. Add two drops of your chosen essential oil to the water bowl, and keep a check that it does not burn dry. Other ways are to add two drops of essential oil to a plant mister full of warm water, and spray the air every few hours, or to add the same amount to a vase or bowl of water placed over a radiator or other heat source. Soak a clean tea-towel in the solution, wring out, and place on a radiator – it will release the fragrance as it dries. Another good idea is to place a few drops on a dry cloth, and use to wipe over light bulbs. When the bulb heats up it will release the fragrance into the room. All of these measures are excellent ways to perfume and change an atmosphere, or to disinfect a sick room.

Essential oils may also be diluted and worn as a perfume, or mixed with an emulsifier and added to the final rinse to delicately fragrance clothes or upholstery. This is especially useful in hot weather, when insect-deterrent oils can be chosen.

Making your own oil blends

When choosing oils for therapeutic use, let their recognized benefits be your guide, but for making your own perfumes and to fragrance your home, follow your nose too.

Oils come in family groupings according to their scent as well as the type of plant they come from. These can be classified as:
- woody (cedarwood, pine, howood)
- herbaceous (marjoram, clary sage)
- citrus (bergamot, lemon)
- floral (rose, geranium)
- resinous (olibanum)
- spicy (ginger, black pepper).

Traditionally, oils blend well with their own and neighbouring groups, e.g. woody and herbaceous, or floral and resinous.

Each blend of oils can be said to have three main components: a top note, a middle note, and a base note. Although the recognition of each note can be fairly subjective because the oils will smell differently to each nose the following can be used as a guideline.

A top note is fresh, with a light quality that evaporates quickly – it is often the first thing that you notice. Oils with a good top note include lemon, eucalyptus and light basil.

A middle note forms the main bulk of the scent – not being immediately apparent behind the top note, it emerges after the first impression. Look for this in lavender, geranium, and marjoram.

A base note is usually fairly rich, and heavy – it is the scent that lingers, usually emerging slowest of all. It fixes and holds the lighter oils, stopping them from dispersing too quickly. Good examples are jasmine, myrrh and patchouli.

Experiment for yourself, and see how well defined your nose can become. You can look more deeply into each oil, and determine whether it has a predominant base note, or is more balanced. Ylang ylang is well balanced in its own right and could sit in any position within a scent blend – it has a sweet, powerful top note that is quite flowery, its middle or second-taste is rich and creamy, and it has a heavy soft, slightly spicy but floral base note.

To wear as a perfume, add three drops of any oil, or oil blend, to a tablespoon of a carrier oil, and apply to the pulse spots on the neck, wrists, and behind the knees. Store in a dark bottle, or make a new blend every day, or every few days, to match your changing moods.

Visiting a practitioner

On consulting an aromatherapist who uses massage, you might expect the initial appointment to last anything up to two hours. This is so that there will be time for you to get to know each other, and for the practitioner to take a brief history from you, as well as giving you a treatment. You may be asked for any relevant medical information, and for more general questions about your feelings and emotions. Certainly your mood that day and any particular aches and pains you might have will assist the practitioner in selecting the appropriate oils.

Once the history is taken you will generally be asked to undress and lie on the massage couch. Some people leave their underwear on, and some undress completely – it is up to you to do whatever feels the most comfortable. The practitioner will be quite used to working with people in various states of undress, modesty is always addressed, and you will be partly covered with towels or a sheet to ensure that you do not become cold.

The aromatherapist should be able to answer any questions you may have about the treatment, and will also take your lead on whether to talk or not during the massage. Some people find they like to relax and be quiet, while others prefer to talk a little. This may also change from massage to massage, depending on your mood.

At the end of the treatment you will have some time to

rest and gather yourself before getting dressed again. The practitioner may then suggest some oils for you to add to your bath water, to use as a room scent, or whatever they feel is appropriate. This is also the time when you can ask any questions, and arrange another appointment. Subsequent visits are likely to be shorter because the practitioner will already have your history or notes, and will usually just want an update on how you are feeling, and what your reaction was to the last treatment.

It is advisable to wear casual clothes, or to take a change of clothes with you because the carrier oils used in the massage can stain some synthetic-mix fabrics (like poly-cottons). Some clinics will have a shower facility, but it is nice to let the oils continue to be absorbed through your skin and to carry the aroma for a while after the treatment – ideally through until the next morning. Aromatherapists can be found at many alternative health clinics, and at some gyms, fitness centres and hair and beauty salons. Some work from home, and you may be lucky enough to find one who will visit your own home, bringing with them a massage couch and a selection of oils. Some aromatherapists advertise in the *Yellow Pages* and in health food shops and similar outlets, but, as with any practitioner, a personal recommendation is by far the best guide.

The oils

There are dozens of oils currently on the market. Some, like jasmine, are very expensive because the amount of oil obtained from each plant is so small, and it needs to be handled very

---

carefully during processing; then of course there are shipping and packaging costs. Other plants, like rosemary, grow in many more parts of the world and yield their oil more easily. Essential oil of rosemary is relatively inexpensive.

The following is a small selection of essential oils that could form the basis of a good kit for home use. Care must always be taken during pregnancy (when some oils are contra-indicated, or could have detrimental side effects) and aroma-therapy should not be used without the advice and monitoring of a healthcare professional.

Oil	Home Uses
Clary sage	This warming, soothing oil is good for the chest, and can be used for massage and in steam inhalations. Use before bedtime to enhance the quality of dreams, and avoid alcohol when using.
Eucalyptus	A strong, clear oil that is used to treat sinuses – a drop on the pillow or on a handkerchief will help easy breathing. Add to steam inhalations and to fragrance a room.
Frankincense	The great rejuvenator. This oil is also very comforting when anxious. It will deepen breathing and can be used in massage or steam inhalations.
Geranium	This refreshes, balances and uplifts. It is a great emotional stabilizer, and can be added to the bath water, or used as a room fragrance.

Howood	A woody, evocative oil that is a strong pelvic decongestant. Add to footbaths, or use to fragrance a room.
Jasmine	This beautiful oil is a strong anti-depressant and mood enhancer. Add to massage oil, baths, and to perfumes and room scents.
Juniper	A kidney tonic that speeds the elimination of toxins. Deeply stimulating, add to bath and footbaths, or for localized massage.
Lavender	Used to balance the system, relaxes, and stimulates immunity. It has a strong analgesic effect, and is antiseptic. Add one drop to teaspoon of water and apply to relieve the pain of insect bites, stings and small burns.
Peppermint	A digestive aid that is cooling and refreshing. Good for settling nausea, and an effective insect repellent.
Rosemary	The oil of remembering – useful to clear mental dullness and for burning on the desk or in the study. Stimulating overall, and a good antiseptic. Aids circulation.
Sandalwood	Sweet and woody, this oil is often used to evoke a meditative atmosphere. Particularly good for mature skins, and for relieving anxiety and nervous tension. Use in massage and in the bath.
Tea tree	An amazing anti-viral, anti-fungal, anti-bacterial oil from Australia. Use in a wash for skin complaints, or add to the bath for an immune boost.

| Ylang ylang | Soothing, sensual and exotic, this oil is a reputed aphrodisiac. Use in perfumes, as a room fragrance, and in baths. |

Add two drops of any essential oil to a bowl of warm water to make a pleasant hand or foot bath. This is a lovely way to absorb the benefits of the oil when a bath is not possible, e.g. during an illness. Consider jasmine to lift the spirits, Juniper to stimulate circulation and tone the kidneys, or rosemary for its strengthening and invigorating effects.

Add three drops of Tea Tree oil to a bath for a strong boost to the immune system. Add three drops of olibanum for a long, reflective soak that will clear old emotions and memories, or bergamot to balance all the body's appetites, and to strengthen the immune system.

Make an aromatherapy massage oil by adding one drop of up to three essential oils to a saucer of a carrier oil. Choose almond, wheatgerm, sesame or peachnut as base oils, and add geranium, bergamot and lavender for a light, energizing and uplifting blend. Black pepper, juniper and rosemary make a warming and stimulating mix. Choose jasmine, rose and ylang ylang for a sultry blend to enhance femininity and feelings of sensuality.

Whatever blend you choose can be used to massage specific areas like the hands and feet, or for a full body treat from a friend or a lover. Steam inhalations are an excellent form of treatment. Adding a few drops of essential oil to the hot water allows the steam to carry the fragrance and its beneficial effects where they are needed. Pour boiling water into a large bowl and add two drops of essential oil before covering it with a towel for an old-fashioned facial steam. Simply put your head over the bowl, and use the towel to keep the steam in place. Choose sandalwood to soften the skin, or geranium for an instant energy lift. Add thyme or eucalyptus to clear sinus complaints, and loosen any chestiness or congestion. This is a wonderful treatment for a cold or cough, and can be repeated two or three times a day. You can use this to fragrance a room by adding the essential oil to a small bowl of boiled water, and placing it by the door or window. Use two drops of lemongrass to fragrance and disinfect a bathroom or sick room. Add two drops of clary sage to a cup of boiled water and place by your bed over night to enhance your dreaming.

Finding out more
Aromatherapy Associates
68 Maltings Place
Bagleys Lane
London SW6 2BY
Tel: 0171 731 8129
Micheline Arcier Aromatherapy
7 William Street
London SW1X 9HL
Tel: 0171 235 3545

Further Reading

Patricia Davis, *Aromatherapy, An A-Z*, C.W. Daniel Company

Nicola Naylor, *Healing with Essential Oils*, Gill & Macmillan

Daniele Ryman, *The Aromatherapy Handbook*, Century.

BODY FORMS

Yoga • Tai Chi • Qi Gong • Ki Aikido

There are many practices which it would be difficult to describe solely as exercise, or martial art, or energetic movement, although they seem to encompass some or all of these descriptions. The body forms provide a way of integrating body and mind, and strengthening their connection. Coming mainly from the East, where such a synthesis is understood, there are many different styles and techniques, and we are discovering more all the time. Among the commonest in the West are Yoga, T'ai Chi, Qi Gong, and Ki Aikido.

These all work to strengthen the life force or vitality as it manifests in the body. This is called Chi (China), Ki or Qi (Pacific rim), and Prana or Manna (Asia). The Chi is felt to be most accessible as it moves through the body along energy pathways or meridians, and many of these forms seek to work directly to stretch or iron out any potential blockages in these channels.

Yoga is often treated as an exercise in the West, although it is really a complete discipline that includes physical, mental and spiritual exercises. This is how it is still practised in the East.

The physical exercises comprise gentle stretches and the holding of postures, accompanied by special breathing exercises. The system can be very useful for certain body types, but care needs to be taken to find a qualified and experienced teacher. Ideally, the physical positions, or assanas, are achieved through a gentle easing and relaxing of the muscles, and careful monitoring is essential to ensure that the postures are right, and that no harm is done. Osteopaths see a number of patients who have tried yoga classes, or yoga postures, without proper training. Being told to 'just go as far as you can' in a large class of people can be an invitation to push oneself into an extreme position that is no good for the body. Proper assessment, guidance and instruction can make this a wonderful system of healthcare.

As a complete discipline, yoga is said to be tremendously empowering and transformational, uniting body, mind and spirit in a single focus, designed to provide a method for living and a tool for life-style change. The practise of the assanas accompanies specific breathing techniques, or pranayama, and deep relaxation and meditation skills, although there are also sexual, karmic and life-style yoga practices. Once learned, the postures, together with the breathing, and often, meditation, can be practised in sequence to build into a personalised daily programme. These are often done first thing in the morning, as a way of preparing for the day ahead. One of the best known yoga moves is, in fact, called 'greeting the sun'.

T'ai Chi is a form of ritualized movement, which is said to work to unite the physical and spiritual planes. To watch an accomplished practitioner is a great joy; there is an elegance about them and an ethereal quality seldom seen in other forms. They appear as if moving through water, as they slowly shift their weight from one foot to the other, while their body and arms move through a range of slow circular movements.

Once learned, these movements seem to flow on their own, and it is said that one does not do T'ai Chi, one *becomes* the movement. All the individual movements require the knees to be slightly bent, so that the centre of gravity is lowered, and the body to be relaxed and fluid. Chi is the Chinese term for vital energy, and in T'ai Chi this is encouraged to move freely within and around the body, generating enormously pleasurable and profoundly beneficial experiences.

T'ai Chi is often called a moving meditation, and is practised by Buddhist monks and nuns. The movements are an excellent exercise for the body, and their gentle nature aids contemplation and relaxation. Based loosely on Taoist principles of balance and harmony, T'ai Chi is practised all over China and can be seen in parks and town squares as people practise 'the form' before work and during lunch breaks. The form is taught in short or long method, and there are different styles, but they all flow with the same grace and ease of movement.

The form is most usually taught in classes or groups, although individual tuition is available. Classes usually begin with some simple warm-up exercises (see pp. 39–40), and **Qi Gong** exercises are often taught too. T'ai Chi can be done almost anywhere, and practitioners find a daily practice is most useful. It is an absolute delight to perform these sequences in the open air on a warm day, adding a sensual pleasure to the experience, but it is fine to do them indoors. It may at first seem strange to consider doing part of an exercise over and over again, and finding each experience to be quite different, but this is the case with T'ai Chi. Once you have had your first lesson, and learned your first movements, you can begin to practise them, and subsequent lessons will build more elements until you have a sequence that is quite complete in itself.

Qi Gong is a range of postures and stretches which strengthen the person and encourage an easing of the meridians, or energy pathways, that network the body. These can be practised on their own as a dramatically effective system of physical healthcare. Warm-up exercises begin every routine, and seek to connect the whole session by being done in between the postural holds as well, in order to loosen up the body and shake out any muscle tensions. (See pp. 39–40)

The stretches each seek to strengthen and tone one pair of organs, or the energy pathway that connects to them. These are very effective, and just a few minutes spent doing the stretches every day will show benefits after about a week. They build into a sequence that will work the entire body.

The postures are simply held for varying lengths of time, and each one will work on a particular pairing of organs, or along an energy pathway that supplies them. It may sound like something that is very easy to do, but holding the postures in the correct way is very demanding, raising the heart rate and really working the muscles that are involved. In the beginning, it is often only possible to hold each position correctly for perhaps one minute at a time.

Qi Gong is taught in groups, often alongside other practices such as T'ai Chi or Ki Aikido. Individual tuition is also available, and this is very useful because of the accuracy that is required to hold the postures correctly. This is one of the most effective and dramatically beneficial exercise systems that I have encountered. It is simple and pleasurable to do, and just 20–30 minutes a day spent working through the routine will have a positive effect on your life within a very short time.

Ki Aikido is a Japanese martial art which focuses on the spiritual development and awareness of the individual.

Physical strength is not necessary in Ki Aikido, because although it is taught as a contact form, the emphasis is on finding ways to use the aggressor's own force against him/herself. Students are encouraged to concentrate on the state of their own energy, and learn techniques to focus on that and harness the momentum of an attack for use as defence.

Students develop an awareness of 'one point'; the physical centre of gravity that is often called hara. This is a point just below the navel and its energetic importance is as the site where the physical and spiritual energies in the body meet. One technique is called 'keeping weight underside'. This is to maintain the sense of being grounded, and is a way of consciously maintaining physical relaxation. If you hold out your arm and try to exert strength to keep it in position, it will gradually become harder to hold, as tiredness takes its toll. It will therefore be potentially easier for another person to move it. If you concentrate on holding it in a relaxed way, aware of your own centre (hara) and the presence of gravity (keeping the weight on the underside) it is harder for somebody else to move it.

Ki Aikido is taught in classes of anything up to 30 students, and they progress through a grading system, signified by the wearing of coloured belts. The highest grade is a black belt. Although it is essentially an art of self-defence, the practitioner's aim is to develop sufficient skill and awareness to make it unnecessary to engage in any form of physical combat. Ki is the Japanese word for life force, 'ai' means union, and 'do' means path or way. The word then, and the practice, incorporates the individual's vital energy into a way of living.

Qi Gong warm-up exercises

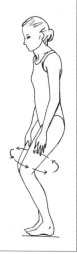

These warm-up exercises are therapeutic in their own right, mobilizing the body and gently opening up the internal energy pathways. Do them once or twice each day for a week to see real benefits in your flexibility and energy levels. They make a good start to the Makka Ho (see pp. 41–3), or any other exercises.

1. Stand with your feet together, and your knees 'soft'. Relax your neck and shoulders, and take a deep breath.

2. Lean forwards slowly, leading with your head, until you can rest your hands loosely on your legs, just above the knees. Bend your

---

knees a little, keeping your feet flat on the floor, and your body straight – as though you were sitting down a little, only there is no chair, so you only drop a small way. This position should feel quite comfortable. Take another breath, and relax your face and shoulders.

3. Keeping your hands in their relaxed hold above your knees, slowly circle your knees around to the left twelve times. Keep your knees together, and your feet flat on the floor. Then circle your knees slowly around to the right twelve times.

4. Relax and stand up straight.

5. Move your feet until they are about shoulder-width apart, and soften your knees as before, letting them bend a little while you keep your back straight, and your neck and shoulders quite relaxed.

6. Take a deep breath, and bring your hands up in front of your heart, then slowly move them straight out in front of you as you breathe out. Pause for just a second, then let your hands

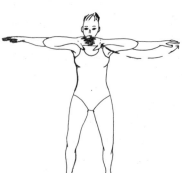

separate, and sweep out around to each side of you, bringing them back in towards your heart as you breathe in. The whole movement is exactly like a breast-stroke manoeuvre. Keep the movement fluid, pausing for just a second as you reach the end of your in and out breaths. Repeat this 15–20 times, then relax, return your hands down to your knees, and stand up straight.

Makka Ho

Makka Ho is a system of exercises to stretch each meridian. It is used by many Shiatsu practitioners. There are six positions that can be performed in sequence to form a complete body workout. Do this every day for about a week to see positive results. Breathe out when moving into and out of each position, and never reach beyond what feels comfortable. Hold each stretch for three deep breaths, and relax further into each stretch with each exhalation.

Stretch 1 – the lungs and large intestine
Stand up with your feet about shoulder-width apart, and your neck and shoulders quite relaxed. Put your hands behind your back, and link your thumbs. Breathe in, and gently stretch your back. Keeping your thumbs linked, breathe out as you slowly swing your arms up and over your head, letting them gently pull your body forward as their weight drops down in front of you. Keep your fingers straight. Take three deep breaths as you hold the stretch, relaxing further into it with each out breath. Slowly and gently uncurl, and return to the starting position. Take a breath, and relax.

Stretch 2 – the stomach and spleen
Kneel down on the floor and sit on your heels with your hands flat on the floor behind you to give you balance. Breathe in, and as you breathe out, slowly raise your hips until you can feel the stretch in the front of your legs. Keep your jaw relaxed, and let your head settle back slightly. Take three deep breaths as you hold the stretch, relaxing further into it with each out breath. Slowly and gently lower your hips and return to your starting position. Take a breath, and relax.

Stretch 3 – The heart and small intestine
Sit on the floor, and keeping your back straight, put the soles of your feet together, and gently pull them in towards you. Breathe in, and as you breathe out take a gentle but secure hold on your toes. Leading with your head, curl your body forwards letting your elbows and knees stretch down to the floor. Let the weight of your elbows carry your knees down as far as they will happily go. Take three deep breaths as you hold the stretch, relaxing further into it with each out breath. Slowly and gently uncurl, and return to your starting position. Take a breath and relax.

Stretch 4 – the kidney and bladder
Sit on the floor with your back straight, and your legs out in front of you. Breathe in and raise your hands up over your head, keeping your back straight, and your feet relaxed. Feel a small stretch in your back. Breathe out, and keeping your back straight, and your head and arms in the same line, gently and slowly relax forward so that your chest drops down towards your knees. Use your eyes to look forward without moving your head. Take three deep breaths as you hold the stretch, relaxing further into it with each out breath. Slowly and gently come back up, and return to your starting position. Take a breath, and relax.

Stretch 5 – the heart protector and triple heater
Sit on the floor with your back straight, and your legs crossed. (If you can sit in the lotus or semi-lotus yoga position, this would be fine.) Cross your arms in front of you, and place them on your knees, palm up. Your right arm will be on your left knee,

and your left arm on your right knee. Take a breath, and as you breathe out, gently stretch forward, keeping your back straight. Feel the stretch in your arms as you aim your forehead towards the floor. Take three deep breaths as you hold the stretch, relaxing further into it with each out breath. Slowly and gently come back up and return to your starting position. Take a breath, and relax.

Stretch 6 – the liver and gall bladder
Sit on the floor with your back straight, and your legs straight and wide apart. Hold the left side of your waist with your right hand, and raise your left hand above your head. Breathe in, and stretch up with your left hand. As you breathe out, stretch down slowly and gently to your right side, aiming your ear to your knee and using your raised arm to help you reach down. Feel the stretch along the side of your body and your legs. Take three deep breaths as you hold this stretch, relaxing further into it with each out breath. Slowly and gently come back up, and return to your starting position. Take a breath and relax.

Finding out more
Iyengar Yoga Institute
223a Randolph Avenue
London W9 1NL
Tel: 0171 624 3080
British T'ai-chi Ch'uan Association and London T'ai-chi Academy
7 Upper Wimpole Street
London W1M 7TD
Tel: 0171 935 8444

Martial Arts Commission
First Floor
Broadway House
15-16 Deptford Broadway
London SE8 4PE
Tel: 0181 691 8711
British Ki Aikido Association
c/o The Secretary,
48 Oakshott Court
Polygon Road
London NW1 1ST
Tel: 0171 281 0877
Community Health Foundation (East–West Centre)
188 Old Street
London EC1V 9BP
Tel: 0171 251 4076
The Lam Clinic
First Floor
70 Shaftesbury Avenue
London WC1V 7DF
Tel: 0831 802 598

Further Reading

Chöygram Trungpa, *The Way of the Warrior*, Shambhala Books

Chungliang Al Huang, *Embrace Tiger, Return to Mountain*, Celestial Arts, USA

Silva, Mira and Shyam Mehta, *Yoga, The Iyengar Way*, Dorling Kindersley

John Stevens, *Aikido The Way of Harmony*, Shambhala Books.

BODYWORK

*Rolfing • Hellerwork • Aston Patterning • Bioenergetics •
Polarity therapy • Reiki or Radiance Technique*

Many physical therapists and healers call themselves bodyworkers. This phrase embraces a range of therapies, and
most often bodyworkers use a synthesis of different techniques they have developed for themselves. In the course
of their training, and with the wide variety of available
workshops, few physical practitioners stick solely to one
particular set of skills.

My own interpretation is of work that is physically
moving and which involves some form of psycho-
emotional content – either a counselling aspect or, more
generally, a body/mind philosophy of which the client is
made aware. In dipping into the reservoir of feelings and
memories that the body holds, all forms of bodywork serve
to remind us of the rich connections that exist between all
parts of ourself.

Bodywork essentially embraces two main types of
therapy – structural bodywork which is concerned with
achieving individual change by focusing on altering or
correcting physical imbalances, and allowing these to
influence the whole person; and body-oriented psychotherapy. This places greater emphasis on the body as a container or manifestation of personal impulses, and seeks to

release emotional and mental blocks from their physical sitings. These distinctions become quite blurred in practice.

The following selection of bodywork styles is representative of the range that is currently available in the West.

Rolfing was devised by Ida Rolf as a way of completely rebalancing the body by realigning any asymmetry. Rolfers work using their hands, elbows or knees to apply deep pressure to the muscles and release them from any habitual or ineffective positioning.

The work involves ten sessions, each usually lasting one hour or slightly longer. Rolfers will begin by assessing the body from all perspectives: sideways, backwards, etc; to get an overall picture of how all the structural elements stack together. Standing in their underwear, the patient or 'Rolfee' will then be photographed. This allows a good before and after comparison to be made, and the Rolfee may have copies of both shots.

Rolfing sessions progress through the body, working on one specific area each time. There can be a degree of pain involved as the Rolfer reaches down deeply into underused or tired muscles. Rolfees are encouraged to express the pain, so yelling and groaning often accompany a session. The effects can be really dramatic – as the before and after photos will affirm, and most people comment on the mental or emotional changes they experience during the ten sessions.

Rolfing has led on to the establishing of several other forms of structurally-aligning bodywork, most notably **Hellerwork**, **Aston Patterning** and **Primal Integration**.

Hellerwork takes a gentler approach to release adhesions in the muscle tissue, and the emphasis is on verbally processing the emotions and thoughts which come up during the bodywork, rather than simply expressing them as a release. Movement education to increase self-awareness is also a facet of this therapy.

Aston Patterning relies more on movement to achieve optimal structural integrity, and is again much gentler on the body than Rolfing. **Postural Integration** unites the Rolfing concept with the ideas of Wilhelm Reich, that a degree of tightness or body 'armour' is a necessary product of developmental and everyday psychological stresses. This allows a more psychotherapeutic element to be brought into the sessions, and enables the mental and emotional releases stemming from the bodywork to be addressed within a treatment.

Bioenergetics is the most established Reichian-based therapy. Reich's theories explore the healing capabilities of the body which he maintained was driven by instinctive or sexual 'life-energies'. He repeatedly asserted the fundamental role of individual sexual energy in continued good health, and encountered much resistance for so doing. A few years before his death in 1957, Reich was imprisoned, ostensibly for ignoring an injunction against his research work, and this is where he died of a heart attack after having all of his books and papers burned.

Dr Alexander Lowen and others refined Reich's basic therapeutic techniques to form bioenergetics, a system that directly addresses any repressed desires and lack of vibrancy or vitality to unite mind, body and energetic process.

Sessions include the client getting into and then holding a number of physical postures, and performing physical exercises, which alongside the use of special breathing techniques, allow stagnant energy to be mobilized or released. The client is encouraged to express the emotions that come up as energy flows through their body. The work alternates between the client perceiving and releasing muscular-emotional blocks, and talking about what is happening, to gain insights as to the nature of the blocks, and their own inner workings.

Grounding and breathing exercises begin each session, to enable the client to focus on their body and really get in touch with it, and these along with many of the other exercises can be practised alone, in between sessions, to continue the work. (See Home Applications, p. 50)

Grounding is about feeling as if you live in your whole body, not just in your head. It is about 'knowing where you stand' in all areas of your life, and 'having your feet on the ground'. It is about embodying your life.

Sessions usually last for one hour, or a little longer, and may be booked as frequently as the client desires. Many people choose to book a few initial sessions quite close together in order to get things moving, and then vary the frequency according to what comes up.

All matter is composed of energy, and some bodyworkers concentrate on the energy of the individual as it manifests in and around their body. There are many different approaches to this work, and healers work with this energy in a variety of ways. (See Healing pp. 113–23)

Polarity therapy uses an interesting type of body map, which views the central energy source, or core of the person, as neutral, and all points beyond that as being either positively or negatively charged. They maintain that the soles of the feet, for instance, are negative poles, and the head is a positive pole; the palm of the left hand having a negative charge, the palm of the right a positive charge. Practitioners use their hands to balance these varying energy states by placing them on the body at prescribed locations.

Reiki or **Radiance Technique** is part of a full system of healthcare that includes dietary and exercise aspects, but in its bodywork requires only a gentle, caring touch. The focus with Reiki is on allowing 'universal energy' into the individual, or helping them to expand so that they may receive it.

These different styles concentrate on working with the individual's own energy, and the energetic exchange with the practitioner or therapist. That this is the focus of the work marks these as distinct from other therapies, but it is worth remembering that all contact, whether physical or not, involves some form of energetic communication. An awareness of this is often what makes the difference and makes for an effective practitioner, whatever style of therapy is used. In any form of bodywork, a sense of, and respect for, the individual's energy is most important, although an exchange does also occur in non-contact therapies.

This bioenergetic-based exercise is one that I use most often because of its simplicity and effectiveness. It is a gentle but powerful introduction to this type of work, and can be practised at any time. It is good for introducing a sense of grounding, and students often tell me that it lets them feel as though 'they really reach to the floor'.

1. Stand in a relaxed way, with your legs slightly apart. Take a deep breath, and as you breathe out, lead with your head and bend forwards as if to touch your toes. Move your weight onto the balls of your feet, and let your upper body relax completely as it hangs down towards the floor. Keep your breathing deep and continuous, not leaving any gaps in it, and allow the rhythm to intensify the experience. Because the hamstring muscles at the back of the thigh are stretched, they may begin to shudder or shake. Encourage this movement, and increase it or magnify it, and keep breathing.

2. It may be that nothing happens beyond a gentle quivering in the muscles, which disappears quite quickly leaving a feeling of great relaxation and warmth in the legs. Sometimes the shaking subsides spontaneously, or it may progress through a sequence of different degrees of movement, throwing up strong memories and feelings as it does so. Allow these to surface, and keep breathing.

The advantage of doing this exercise in a session is that whatever feelings or thoughts come up can be expressed and worked on with the practitioner. When doing this on your own, it is a good idea to process the material in some way for yourself — either write it down, draw it, talk to someone about it, or find some other way to work with it. Your body will just have released a precious piece of information that it needs to have recognised and honoured, so find some way to integrate this experience into your life.

Finding out more
Rolf Institute
80 Clifton Hill
London NW8 0JT.
Tel: 0171 328 9026
Institute of Bioenergetic Medicine
103 North Road,
Parkstone
Poole
Dorset BH14 0LU
Tel: 01202 733762
Polarity Therapy Association U.K.
11 The Lea Allesley Park
Coventry CV5 9HY
Tel: 01203 670847
Radiance Education Unlimited (Reiki)
P.O. Box 1013
London NW3 3LW
Tel: 0171 586 2980

Further Reading

Don Johnson, *The Protean Body: A Rolfer's View of Human Flexibility*, HarperCollins
Alexander Lowen, *Bioenergetics*, Penguin
Alexander Lowen and Leslie Lowen, *The Vibrant Way to Health: A Manual of Bioenergetic Exercises*, Harper and Row.

CHINESE FACE READING AND TONGUE DIAGNOSIS

There is growing interest in this method of diagnosis which originates from Eastern healthcare philosophies and forms an important part of traditional Chinese medicine.

Careful observation of the face and tongue can point towards the condition of the whole body in much the same way as iridologists and reflexologists look to the eyes and to the feet. It is particularly useful in that it requires no tools or techniques, and with the aid of only a mirror can become a useful way of assessing one's own state of health.

We use facial diagnosis all the time, in a small way, whenever we look at another and recognize that they're looking pale, or have been crying, or have good colour in their cheeks. This has simply been developed, and a map of the body imposed upon the colour judgements which we make naturally. It makes such good sense to 'read' this wholly accessible part of the body and many practitioners do so to make a preliminary diagnosis, or confirm findings; it's easy and straightforward, and requires little effort on the part of the patient.

The skin colour, condition and texture are all taken into consideration, alongside an assessment of the features and any particular markings. The face is divided into areas relating to the internal organs and body systems. Their state can then be assessed according to the type of marking or degree of colour present in each area. One clear example of this is the area under the eyes which is said to relate to the kidneys. This is a site which can become puffy when we are retaining water, and which shows when we have been drinking more than a usual amount of alcohol – in the slightly darker than usual bags or rings.

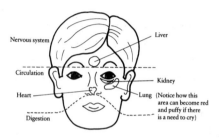

General areas and markings for facial diagnosis

Different races obviously have different basic skin colours, but the colour characteristics of any imbalance remain the same, although practice is needed to discern them. The presence of white spots, for example, can point to an an excess of dairy food in the diet, whereas a general greyish colouring can indicate an under-active liver. This is most common in Western, industrialized countries where the liver is under enormous additional pressure from environmental pollutants and high levels of food additives.

Skin texture may be assessed as rough, oily, dry, wet, etc. Rough skin can result from an excess of saturated fats in the diet, which makes extra work for the liver and kidneys. Dry skin may be caused by higher than usual cholesterol levels or, conversely, by a lack of oil and fat-soluble vitamins.

As a general rule, sore, dry or red skin indicates a condition of internal heat, whereas clammy or moist skin usually points to a colder constitution. These factors are important in terms of diagnosing and treating any illnesses that the patient may manifest. They conform to the Chinese system of analysing most situations as either yin (cold) or yang (hot). This is similar to the diagnosis Shiatsu practitioners make of kyo (empty) or jitsu (full). These terms can apply to all areas of life, where the yang principle would be experienced as expansive, light-giving, masculine, etc., and the yin principle as contracting, dark, feminine, etc. All things may be seen as having a predominance of yin or yang, and the balance between these opposites is perhaps best illustrated by the well-known symbol which incorporates both within the wholeness of the circle.

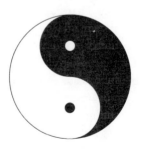

Yin and Yang

An important factor to notice is that within each half is the seed of its opposite. This is where the picture of health diagnosis becomes more complicated, and judgements need to be made as to whether a symptom is full or empty. It can also lead towards the cure when we remember that within each symptom, or illness, or condition, lies the seed of its opposite.

Once this condition is ascertained, the appropriate dietary, exercise and lifestyle changes can be introduced. People with an excess of yin will tend to feel cold, for example, and respond well to warming spices added to the diet, whereas this is the thing to avoid for those with an excess of yang.

The size, shape, positioning and symmetry of features on the face are also of great importance. Eyebrows, for instance, can be classified as close together, far apart, upward or downward slanting, peaked, etc., all reflecting

Left
Paternal influences

Right
Maternal influences

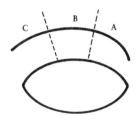 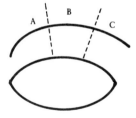

A = Early development, either foetal or youth
B = Mid-part of development, either foetal or middle age
C = Late part of development, either foetal or old age

different constitutional types. Overall, they are said to show the condition of the nervous, digestive, respiratory, circulatory and excretory systems, so they can reveal constitutional states developed during gestation as well as current conditions. The left brow is said to reflect the paternal, and the right brow the maternal influences, and they are further divided to indicate stages of development. The thickness of eyebrow hair shows the degree of basic vitality and can also demonstrate strength of character (an interesting implication for those who pluck their brows!).

The lips relate to the digestive system and the sexual organs (consider a moustache!). The lower lip serves as an indicator for the intestines, the upper lip for the stomach and genitals. A slightly swollen lower lip may indicate constipation, and crust formation in the corners of the mouth may result through difficulties with fat metabolism.

The tongue is a good indicator of overall health, and this can be easily seen if you look at your own tongue every morning. Comparing its colour and degree of coating through good health, periods of ill health and 'mornings after'. This can prove very revealing, confirming how well the body is working. The coating is generally a sign that the body is detoxifying or cleansing itself, and liver function (the main organ of detoxification) can be observed along the sides of the tongue.

The tongue's colour, shape, movements and markings are all important indicators of overall health, and will provide a wealth of information to an experienced practitioner. The colour can range from pale red, its normal state, to deep red, blue and purple, and this usually indicates some level of heat or cold imbalance. Reading the tongue in this way can provide a clear and unambiguous diagnosis when there are conflicting symptoms, or a complicated health picture. The coating on the tongue also yields important information, and the practitioner will assess its colour, thickness, texture, moisture levels and how easy it is to scrape off. A healthy tongue will be seen to have a thin white coating, but this can change according to what you eat, and the seasons. The effects of some medications show very clearly in the tongue's coating, e.g. antibiotics will cause it to peel.

The different areas of the tongue are held to correspond to different organs of the body. The tip is the heart; the band immediately behind that the lungs. In the central area, moving to the rear of the mouth, first comes the spleen, then the stomach. On your right side is the gall bladder, and on your left the liver. And across the furthest back portion of the tongue, in order, are the intestines, bladder then kidneys.

Cracks in the tongue are believed to be caused by 'the drying up of body fluids', and indicate some form of Chi deficiency in the area to which they relate. A crack in the middle of the tongue along the central line points to a lowered stomach energy, and cracks running across the tongue indicate lowered kidney energy.

The tongue, like the skin on the face, also shows the passage of time quite distinctly, and ageing with a depletion of energy shows itself in cracks across the surface.

In keeping with its Chinese origins, some facial signs are also said to indicate the energetic state of the organ or body part to which they relate. This can then point to imbalances or difficulties before they manifest physically.

To this end, many emotional states and vitality observations can be made by an experienced practitioner.

It is well worth taking another look at people's faces; observing, for instance, the size and positioning of the ears (high placement is said to indicate intelligence); and the depth of the lines connecting the nose to the corners of the mouth – the career lines. More practitioners are now using this form of diagnosis as an aid in determining the condition and the progress of their patients, and as a useful way of involving the patient in the process of their own healthcare.

On a personal level, it can be used to provide an immediate reference – pointing to periods of excess or undernourishment, and as an aid to understanding how to maintain energy levels. Although professional assistance is needed to accurately diagnose constitutional states and any disease process, a thorough look at your face using this method can prove beneficial on an everyday level.

Yang foods, such as grains, pulses, sea vegetables and fish can be added to the diet if extra concentration or concerted effort is required for a short period of time. Yin foods – leafy green vegetables, fruits, and salads generally – can then help you wind down afterwards. It is well worth experimenting with these simple, effective dietary measures.

Finding out more
Neal's Yard Therapy Rooms
Mark Reidy, Lic. Ac.
Neal's Yard
Covent Garden
London WC2H 9DP
Tel: 0171 379 7662
Community Health Foundation
188 Old Street
London EC1V 9BP
Tel: 0171 251 4076

Further reading

Dylana Accolla with Peter Yates L.Ac., *Back to Balance*, Newleaf
Michio Kushi, *Your Face Never Lies*, Avery
Giovanni Maciocia, *Tongue Diagnosis in Chinese Medicine*, Eastland Press.

CLAY THERAPY

Clay is used extensively by many naturopaths, and may be taken internally in liquid form, or used externally in a pack applied to the skin. The rich mixture of minerals that the clay contains will determine its colour and consistency. It has strong attractive qualities that make it particularly helpful in speeding up the elimination of toxins and poisons from the body.

Mixed into a paste with a good quality vegetable oil, it can be applied to the skin as a soother, and is used to treat a variety of irritated skin complaints. The addition of two drops of ti tree essential oil makes it a very effective external treatment for fungal conditions like athlete's foot, and adding two drops of lavender essential oil helps soothe and calm the skin still further.

The paste can be applied as a poultice over a very small area – to draw out a boil, for instance, or as a body pack covering up to 70 per cent of the skin surface, for more widespread conditions. In acute situations, e.g. a widespread allergic reaction of the skin, the paste can be painted on almost all over before bed, and rinsed away the following morning. Used this way it can also help relieve sleeplessness and night-time scratching, as well as improving the condition of the skin.

Taken internally as a drink, clay is especially useful in light cases of heavy metal or fungal poisoning. Many people take it on a regular basis for its blood cleansing qualities, and its role in increasing the oxygen content of the blood. Clay does contain aluminium, and although this does not leak into the system, its long-term internal use is nevertheless not recommended in old age, pregnancy, or in immune-compromised individuals.

Clay can also be used as a cleansing agent in place of soap or shampoo, and this is especially useful in the presence of any contact allergies, and for irritated skin. An effective cleanser, clay does not challenge normal skin pH or acidity.

For the use of clay in modelling and as a medium of expression see Self-Expression (pp. 270–1).

A clay poultice is a useful treatment for boils, ulcers and infections, but it is also good for back pain, and decalcification (due to its high mineral content) to relieve arthritic conditions and inflammations.

To make a clay poultice for use on small parts of the body:
1. Place two tablespoons of powdered clay in a pottery bowl or dish, and cover with spring or bottled water. Leave to soak for about two hours, and then mix into a smooth paste using a wooden spoon. (Do not use metal because the clay will absorb it.)

   2. Spoon the paste about half an inch thick onto the middle

---

of a strip of cotton cloth or a bandage, and apply directly to the skin. Use the long dry ends to tie it in place. Leave the poultice on for a minimum of two hours. You can replace this up to three times a day, and the prepared paste can be kept in a bowl for up to three days, so long as it is kept moist, and is carefully covered so as not to absorb any odours.

To prepare a clay drink

Drinking clay water is particularly detoxifying and cleansing. It can be useful after episodes of over-indulgence in rich foods and alcohol, or as part of a detox programme. To take as part of a cleansing programme, drink it every morning for about three weeks, and follow with one week off. This is best undertaken during the spring and autumn when it can complement other detox plans, but it can be used at any time of year.

1. Before going to bed, add one teaspoon of powdered clay to a glass of spring or bottled water, and mix it with a wooden spoon. Leave overnight to settle, and in the morning drink the water and throw away the clay. Wait half an hour before eating or drinking anything else.

Take this every day for about three weeks, and then have one week's rest before continuing the treatment, if desired.

Further Reading

Raymond Dexteric, *The Healing Power of Clay*, Vivre en Harmonie, France
Harry Lindlahr, *Natural Therapeutics*, C.W. Daniel Company.

COUNSELLING

Counselling can take many forms depending upon the counsellor's training and the individual's reasons for seeking this type of support. Most usually it will address a particular issue or difficulty, and last for a relatively short period of time. These are the main differences between it and the psychotherapies, which generally require a longer term commitment to working in a much wider context (See Talking Therapies pp. 301–7). To muddy this distinction, however, there is also psychological or psychotherapeutic counselling, which works at a deep level with the individual's own process.

People often seek out a counsellor for advice or support in much the same way that the advice of elders or wise men and women would be sought in other societies. The North American Indians have a tradition of seeking this wisdom from their ancestors, or from the Shamans which are common in this and other cultures.

Counselling for specific situations is clearly labelled – health counselling or bereavement counselling for example, where people with these difficulties may find comfort, help and someone to listen. The initial session is an opportunity for both people to see whether they want to work with each other, and is the time to determine precisely what is needed, and what the counsellor can provide. It may be that practical advice is sought, or, as is often the case, that what is really wanted is somebody who will listen, without judging.

An enormous benefit provided by a counsellor is their objectivity – they may have, and voice, their own opinions, but there is no existing relationship or history between counsellor and client. There is also the security of knowing that whatever is discussed in a session will be completely confidential.

This discretion enables people to explore issues fully in a safe environment, before integrating them into their lives. It may be that the counsellor is used as a sounding board, to try out new ways of relating; or as an important source of support during times of change.

The techniques used in a session will depend on the counsellor's training as well as the individual's reasons in seeking out this form of help. Two basic types of skills are employed – directive or active counselling and a more receptive approach. The latter builds on the work of Carl Rogers, who developed a style known as client-centred therapy. He maintained that the only frame of reference that could be of any use to a client would be one which they built themselves. In practice, this means that the focus of the work is in defining and clarifying the client's own understanding and resources. Counsellors working in this way will mirror the client; on the simplest level often repeating or simply rephrasing what they hear, and offering it back to the client.

This is a very good technique for use in times of distress,

when we are often unable to take in advice or new ideas and will respond best to a validation of our own feelings. It can make us feel very secure, and more willing to open up about ourselves and our concerns. It is also extremely useful for encouraging confidence in one's own thoughts and ideas and in increasing feelings of self-esteem.

More directive approaches include those working within a particular framework – such as psychological astrologers. They have information to impart as well as the offer of a new perspective or framework within which to view both the current situation and developmental factors. Psychic counsellors also work actively, translating what they perceive of, or in, a person in an effort to give them as much pertinent information, and therefore as great a choice, as possible. Visits to both psychological astrologers and psychic counsellors are likely to be on an irregular basis, or even as 'one-offs'.

Although the basics of all counselling sessions are the same – the client and the practitioner both talk to each other; sometimes over a desk, sometimes on a sofa in a sitting-room type situation – that is really where the similarity ends. It is important to establish what you are looking for as early as possible in your search for somebody to work with. You may also need to be prepared to visit a number of different counsellors before finally deciding on one.

Sometimes you will establish a rapport immediately, or have a positive gut feeling that this is the person you want to work with. In order for the sessions to be as productive as possible, you will need to find someone whom you feel you can trust, and who you feel understands you. If particular things are important to you in your choice of counsellor, perhaps sexual orientation, or political awareness, then it is appropriate to ask this of them in the same way as you might enquire as to their experience in the field, or any areas of special interest that they might have.

Sessions usually last for between 50 minutes and an hour, and their frequency will usually be agreed during the first or second visit. In the case of couples counselling, where both partners are seeking assistance together, this may take longer to establish. In some instances it may be appropriate to agree to a fixed number of appointments, perhaps four or six, and then to reassess the situation. This provides an opportunity to get on and tackle a specific area of difficulty at the same time as allowing the counselling relationship to develop.

Counsellors usually take their clients by referral from other practitioners, although some also advertise in specialist journals and locally at Citizens Advice Bureaux, etc. This usually happens when a counsellor is just beginning their work.

The training colleges keep registers of their graduates, and those offering long courses will sometimes encourage students to begin work before they qualify; they then work for a reduced fee and should get good supervision from their tutors or course supervisors. Details of specific counsellors – for debt, bereavement, etc. – can be found at most local libraries and CAB offices.

Finding out more
The British Association for Counselling
37A Sheep Street
Rugby
Warwickshire
CV21 3BX
Tel: 01788 78328/9
Irish Association of Counselling and Therapy
8 Cumberland Street
Dun Laoghaire
Co. Dublin
Tel: 01 230 0061
Centre for Counselling and Psychotherapy Information
21 Lancaster Road
Notting Hill
London W11 1QL
Tel: 0171 221 3215
Relate (formerly Marriage Guidance Council)
Local addresses in the telephone directory
Faculty of Astrological Studies
396 Caledonian Road
London N1
Tel: 0171 700 3556

Further Reading

W. Dryden et al (eds), *Handbook of Counselling in Great Britain*, Routledge
S. Quilliam and I. Grove-Stephenson, *The Counselling Handbook*, Thorsons, 1990.

CRANIO-SACRAL THERAPY
AND CRANIAL OSTEOPATHY

These two distinct therapies stem from the same roots, and both maintain that it is the slight and almost imperceptible movements of the body that can generate well-being, or be implicated in disease and disharmony. Cranial osteopaths follow a strong structural model and mostly limit their work to the bones of the skull, Cranio-sacral therapists, as the name implies, use a more functional model, and will work throughout the body.

There are a number of bones in the head – in a baby these are separate, to allow some contraction as they move through the birth canal. The fontanelles which are evident at birth are the potential spaces for the bones should they be needed. As the baby gets older, these fontanelles disappear from sight as the bones grow closer together, the joins between the bones, however, remain potentially mobile throughout life.

Both therapies agree that a number of health difficulties can be traced back to the birth process and the first few months of life, and the release of any obstructions felt between the bones of the skull can be tremendously beneficial. This is particularly so if forceps or suction techniques were used. It is becoming increasingly common for

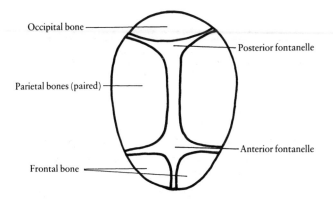

The foetal skull seen from above

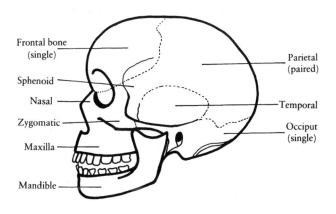

Mobile bones of adult skull, side view

cranio-sacral therapists to be present at a birth, or to treat both mother and baby immediately afterwards.

Cranio-sacral therapy is an exquisitely gentle yet profoundly effective method for treating the whole body and effecting structural change. Although called cranial, the techniques are used throughout the body, and often involve some form of direct contact with the patient's energy field. The release of holding patterns within the body may also allow emotions to surface and become conscious. The gentle nature of the work makes it particularly helpful in the treatment of newborn babies, older people, those in pain, and in any situations where more physically based treatments would be inappropriate.

Developed in the early 1900s by the pioneering work of an American osteopath, William G. Sutherland, these 'new' therapies are in fact steeped in ancient tradition and healing lore. Some of the earliest pictorial records of healing show a simple 'laying on of hands' and written evidence tells of 'the art of listening'. This is the essence of cranio-sacral work. The practitioner uses their hands to listen to, or feel, the intrinsic movement patterns of the person; and employs simple techniques to magnify or lead the body into releasing and rebalancing itself.

Sutherland investigated the structural links between different areas of the body. He developed a theory that the bones of the skull could, by their positioning, affect and be affected by other areas of the body. To substantiate this, he began his work by developing a type of American football-helmet with chunks of movable padding. He experimented on himself by using the helmet to limit the movement of specific cranial bones, and carefully noted his physical and emotional responses. He soon discovered that areas as distant as his toes could be affected by the immobilization of these bones, and charted a host of emotional reactions also. His wife has written a touching account of what it was like living with him during this time – in particular not knowing what sort of a person he would be from one day to the next.

Sutherland then went on to work with the soft tissues and fascial arrangements of the body, and developed his theories further to include an appreciation of the body's subtle structural integrity and movement patterns. He noted that all the bones of the body display an almost imperceptible movement, and discovered the key sites where interruption of such movements or blockages could be relieved.

This work was further developed by Dr Randolph Stone, who expanded some of Sutherland's concepts, and in the 1960s and 1970s by Dr John Upledger, who synthesized the techniques into a full-body approach. The prime source of this inner motion is the process of cerebro-spinal fluid (CSF) production and reabsorption.

CSF is a viscous, jelly-like substance produced by the brain which provides protection for it and the spinal cord. It bathes and envelops the system, encased by the meninges and the bony protection of the bones of the head and spine. If the brain were a precious gift, CSF would be the packing material, the meninges a cling-film coating to hold it all together, and the bones would be the presentation box.

The movement of the CSF can be perceived through an experienced touch, and its rhythms and patterns of motion yield a wealth of information as to the condition of the whole body. Other body movements can also be felt in this way – the sway of all the bones in response to breathing; the waves of peristalsis moving through the gut; even the minute, fluid motions of the organs themselves. Connecting with these rhythms and bringing them to the patient's awareness is often enough in itself to effect change.

Treatment is a deeply relaxing experience, enabling the patient to still their conscious mind and place their attention on their own inner resources. Feeling only the weight, or even gentler touch, of the therapist's hands, they can perceive subtle inner changes. Becoming aware of alterations in internal pressure, movements and releases of energy is often accompanied by changes in breathing patterns (the breath may slow down, or become deeper), or stomach gurgles – a good sign of relaxation.

People will often be aware of what is occurring in one part of their body while the therapist's hands are placed some distance away. This is due to the continuity of fluids and fascias (a sort of inner skin for the muscles and organs) throughout the body; everything is connected. Most often, as the treatment progresses, the patient becomes more and more relaxed, and the therapist's touch almost imperceptible. People often describe their feelings as those of actually being inside their own bodies, or of being in touch with their own energetic state; losing the sense of being separated from the world by their skin. This can lead to mystical, religious or 'peak' experiences.

Cranio-sacral therapy is often used as a technique for personal growth, in the great understanding and insights it can provide. It is tremendously effective on a physical level too; in its gentleness it can be used for structural change when the body is in too much pain to allow an osteopathic adjustment, and its depth allows it to access long-term or deep-seated physical difficulties.

Most cranial workers are osteopaths who have studied cranio-sacral techniques as post-graduates, although some people take the route from another form of healing. The advantage of an osteopathic training is the thorough knowledge of anatomy and physiology, and an understanding of the laws of mechanics as applied to the body. They will also have a greater knowledge of general pathology. All of these can be learned, however, and those coming to the work without manipulative concepts may be more open to its subtler aspects.

Treatments usually take place with the patient lying on a treatment couch and fully relaxed, although some techniques need the patient to be seated. Sessions last an hour, on average, and there will often be time after the treatment to discuss the therapist's findings, and the patient's perceptions. This is particularly important if the patient has experienced the work at a deep level, as they may need to talk about their experience and any implications on an emotional or spiritual level. Sometimes, of course, the treatment is almost exclusively physical, in which case the time may be used for postural advice or ongoing care details.

Without detailed anatomical knowledge it is hard to experience this for yourself at home, but one of the cranio-sacral techniques that is often used is a way of gauging the symmetry of movement throughout the body. Although diagnostic in nature, contacting the body's rhythmic pulsing at this level is deeply relaxing, and the skills needed to go within oneself, into a quiet, receptive and almost meditative state, are richly rewarding. Your experience of this should be one that is calming, quieting and relaxing.

1. Sit in a comfortable position where you will not be disturbed, and keep your spine straight and your feet flat on the floor. Gather a number of cushions or pillows around you. Close your eyes, and get a sense of where your body is now – how relaxed and symmetrical it is, and how easy it feels in this position. Now use your hands to rest on the top of your thighs with your fingers pointing straight down towards your knees. Use the cushions or pillows to support your elbows so that your hands and arms can relax completely.

2. Close your eyes again, and imagine yourself using your hands to tune in to the movement patterns that your legs are making. Picture yourself concentrating, as if you were listening with your hands, and they were conveying the information to your thinking brain.

3. It may take a little time for you to concentrate your awareness sufficiently, but you will soon feel some movement in your thighs. This is usually gentle, and quite minute – when you start to follow it, it may slip away from you. Persevere through leaving your hands and your awareness just waiting, and the rhythm and the movement will return. They are often like a slight rolling motion, and as you stay with them you will notice slight differences between each leg, and between the in and out movements on each side. Do not be surprised if the

movements and their quality or frequency change while you are tuning in to them in this way. If this is the first time that you have listened to your body in any way, it may well be a profound and moving experience, it is certainly always exciting to discover what is going on beneath your hands.

4. When you are ready, free this deep connection and slowly withdraw your awareness, even though your hands are still lying in a relaxed way on top of your thighs. Leave them there for a short while, and think through the experience.

You can repeat this with your arms by resting each hand on the other forearm, with the fingers pointing straight up towards the elbows. You will need to rest your elbows on pillows again. Feeling your body's movements in this way is deeply relaxing and enjoyable, and it is also healing, because any direct contact with these deep inner rhythms has a beneficial effect upon them. You may indeed notice changes after you have performed this exercise – often my students talk of feeling looser or easier around the joints, or of being more flexible and experiencing ongoing relaxation.

Do this as often as you choose, for its positive effects on your body, or to deepen your communication with your body-self. Consider developing your experience further by consulting a cranio-sacral practitioner.

Finding out more
Cranial Osteopathic Association
478 Baker Street
Enfield
Middlesex EN1 3QS
Tel: 0181 367 5561
Karuna Core Therapies
Curtisknowle House
Curtisknowle, near Totnes,
Devon TQ7 7JX
Tel: 0154 882 583
The Upledger Institute
11211 Prosperity Farms Road
Palm Beach Gardens
Florida 33410, USA
Tel: (800) 223 5880

Further Reading

Harold Magoun, *Osteopathy in the Cranial Field*, Journal Printing Co., Missouri
Adah Sutherland, *With Thinking Fingers*, Cranial Academy, Kansas City
John E. Upledger, DO FAAO and John D. Vredovoogd MFA, Seattle, *Craniosacral Therapy*, Eastland Press.

CYCLES AND SEASONS

Just as nature works its way through the seasons of the year, so natural cycles have a deep impact on our lives. Many different healthcare philosophies have their own daily timetables, and will plot to the hour the ebb and flow of our physical energy. We can embrace for ourselves the workings of nature, and learn to follow our own inner cycles and seasons. Eating in harmony with the time of year, and often just looking around at what the world is doing outside our windows, are ways of getting in touch with this great timetable.

The moon exerts an enormous influence on our bodies, as well as on the planet, as our water levels respond to its magnetic pull. This monthly cycle is mirrored in women's own menstrual rhythm. The sun, too, makes itself felt within our bodies, as its mid-day strength resonates with our own digestive fire, drawing it to a peak at noon. Respecting these instinctive responses allows us to feel more at ease with ourselves and more relaxed physically. Simple measures, like marking menstruation with some form of retreat or ceremony rather than letting it pass unnoticed, mean that we can honour what is sacred in our lives and foster a greater integrity between our physical responses and our general awareness.

Spiritual teachings speak of the spiral or cyclic nature of our journey through life, and of the continuous cycle of death and rebirth. At our smallest observable level of atomic distribution, spirals and cycles are again evident in the matrix of physical matter. They recur endlessly throughout our lives as symbols and teachers, and in the reality of our daily lives. Learning to recognize these recurring patterns and to live in harmony with them, enables us to relax into a secure system that is comforting and life enriching, providing a strong structure for our everyday needs. Physically, everything about us from the rhythm of our breathing to the function of our immune system, follows its own life cycle. When we are active during the day, and rest to rejuvenate and replenish ourselves at night, we are living out one of our more basic life cycles. We can see the growth cycle of our skin, hair and nails most clearly of all, and witness what always seems like a miracle when small cuts and abrasions simply disappear as the injured layers of skin are replaced with new ones. This regeneration is occurring all over our bodies all the time, fuelled by the energy we take in, and using the material from the foods that we eat, and following the blueprint from our genes. Almost every cell in your body can renew itself, and over the course of your lifetime, will do so many times.

One strikingly effective way to co-ordinate all the elements of our own lives is to imagine them as points on a wheel of health, which rolls along through the course of our time here. On the outside of the circle, or the rim of the wheel, is room for all the aspects, directions, drives and energies that fill your world, and there is room for those that you want to have in it. Your place is in the centre. Ask yourself what you would need in order to return to that place of complete balance right now. Look from there to see which element is lacking, or too dispersed, and is causing your wheel to wobble, and which element is present or repeated to too great a degree and is reinforcing the buckling. Ask yourself these questions regularly, and let your answers guide you towards greater understanding and enjoyment of your health.

You can plot your day according to a sense of balance, in order to achieve harmony between all of your commitments. Spending eight hours of each day in your own service, eight hours doing something for others, and eight dedicated to rest and renewal allows most needs to be met.

The seasons have an effect on every area of our lives, from how we feel physically, to the way we respond emotionally. Sometimes, just looking out at the weather can reinforce what is going on in our inner world. It is seductively easy to feel some lethargy and laziness when we are in the middle of spring rains, and the world seems damp, grey and lifeless. A cold, blustery winter day does nothing to encourage us to linger out of doors and enjoy a casual stroll, and who wants to remain inside when summer is reaching its peak, and the busy-ness of nature can be felt in the air all around. We can remember this when our inner climate becomes listless or cold, or when it seems to burst forth without heed to anything other than the time of year.

Balance your body's nutritional needs by eating with the seasons to ensure optimum vitality. Spring makes available to us a wealth of new shoots and green salad vegetables, and is the ideal time to follow some type of cleansing routine based on detoxifying foods. (See Detox pp. 88–90) The summer sees more fruits and vegetables become available, and we receive nutrition from the lengthened daylight hours and from our contact with the elements as we follow our natural inclinations to spend more time out of doors. Autumn sees us gathering in the harvest, and starting to use more grains along with the richness of other vegetables and fruits. This is another useful time for cleansing, in preparation for the winter months ahead. During the winter we rely more upon our stores – of grain and vegetables, and there is little new growth except for the root vegetables, which grow deep down in the ground.

We can prepare our foods using seasonal values too – using long, slow, oven cooking to mirror the conditions root vegetables thrive in, and to gather and store the energy within them to keep us warm in winter. Spring lends itself towards stir-frying and other fast methods of cooking that retain the colour and texture of the foods themselves.

Ayurveda, the system of natural healthcare that comes from Asia, suggests the following timetable to foster optimum health and vitality, and ensure that all your body's physical needs are met. This includes time for yoga or other gentle exercise, meditation, and self-massage – all elements that we in the West need to include in our routines to help us balance our busy lifestyles.

6–8am
Rise
Wake a little before sunrise each day, to enjoy the dawn and to let your day be filled with the sense of lightness, exhilaration and freshness that fills this hour of the morning. Ideally you should wake up without being jarred by the sound of an alarm. The busy morning schedule of self-care requires a little more time than we are used to, but there is much to do to get the body off to a good start. Ayurveda recommends that you massage your body with warmed sesame oil before bathing, and if this is not possible for any reason, then at least the head and the feet should be massaged. Then there is time to exercise and meditate before breakfast.

Noon–1pm
Lunch
This marks the next major landmark in the day, and the time when the digestive fire is burning at its strongest. This is when to have the main meal of the day, and to give yourself time to digest it before moving on to other things. Taking five minutes to rest after eating is sufficient, and a gentle walk afterwards will aid the process.

6–7pm
Dinner
The end of the working day is marked with an opportunity for more meditation or a second brief walk, before preparing for the evening meal. Having eaten the main meal of the day at noon, dinner is more moderate, and can again be followed by a few minutes rest, and a short walk.

9.30–10.30pm

Bedtime

After an evening of light activity, an early night means being able to get up early the next day. Avoid anything too stimulating, like action-packed TV late in the evening, and develop a restful routine in preparation for bed to calm and soothe you.

If this timetable is light years away from your own routine, consider adopting it for a week to see whether it makes any difference to your energy levels. The most noticeable effect I see is from taking such an early night – it truly does seem to balance the quality of energy throughout the day, and removes the common mid-afternoon slump more effectively than any other measure I know. It can be quite a revelation to many people that looking after their body is something that is worth scheduling time for, and even getting up earlier to do. If you do this, however, the respect and the time commitment pay dividends in terms of renewed vitality and the easing of minor health concerns, as well as in the renewed energy and vitality that follow.

Further Reading

Ricard Adams and Max Hooper, *Nature through the Seasons*, Penguin

Deepak Chopra, MD, *Perfect Health: The Complete Mind/Body Guide*, Bantam

Johanna Paungger and Thomas Poppe, *Moon Time*, C. W. Daniel Company.

DETOXIFICATION

This is something that your body is doing all the time. The elimination of toxins through a variety of routes enables the body to function properly and ensures good health. Naturopathy, along with many other natural health philosophies, maintains that it is this process of clearing out the body that facilitates good health, and that disease is a natural result of a failure to eliminate toxins, or a break down of the body's eliminative routes.

A clear example of this is the bowel. Irritable-bowel conditions, cancers and a host of other gut disturbances are most common in societies with a high intake of refined foods. When these are eaten at the expense of the natural roughage, which is to be found in fruits and vegetables, the walls of the colon can become clogged and ineffective. This means not only a lowering of the rate of absorption of nutrients from the foods we eat, but can also result in some substances remaining in the gut for years!

There are a number of avenues available for such elimination. The liver does much of the work of filtering substances within the body, and these can be expelled through the work of the kidneys; in urine, through the skin, by perspiration, the lungs and mucous membranes, and the bowel. The efficient functioning of all routes is necessary to full health. You can see this clearly for yourself when a period of constipation is accompanied by spots or pimples appearing on the skin, or in the obvious fluid bloating the morning after larger than usual alcohol intake.

The body is continuously producing substances which need to be expelled – every muscle activity, chemical process and stage of growth leads to an amount of unnecessary by-products or debris. Each hormonal, emotional, and energetic response creates substances which the body needs to be rid of. And most of the chemicals we ingest through the foods we eat, the air we breathe and the substances we contact have no place at all inside our system.

There are a number of measures we can take to ensure that our eliminative routes and organs are functioning as well as they can. Dry skin brushing (see Skincare p. 285) and good personal hygiene aid skin function, and drinking adequate amounts of fresh, clean water helps the kidneys work well. Diet is one of the most effective ways of clearing the bowel, and can also allow time for the whole body to cleanse itself. Eating foods that are as close as possible to their natural state releases a large amount of energy for use within the body. When we simplify the job of digestion, we liberate the huge amounts of energy that are usually used to discern, process and progress foodstuffs. This energy can then be used to concentrate on detoxification and any other healing work that is needed.

Nature provides us with obvious times to detoxify. Each change of season marks a transition from one form of behaviour to another, the range of foods which is naturally and locally available to us alters as do the ways we spend our time, and the body changes its rate of metabolism.

This transition period is a time to use diet to support the whole system – making life as simple as possible so that the body's own vitality can control its resources and do whatever work is necessary.

If we look at the foods which are naturally available, we can see some times of the year being more abundant than others. Harvest time in autumn has traditionally been a time of feasting; late winter, before the first spring shoots appear, a time of fast. Women have their own inner 'seasons' as we move through our own monthly cycle.

There are detox diets which last for a month or more, and these give the body an opportunity for a thorough cleansing, and give good support to the immune system. Spending just a few days on simple foods can be useful too, or one day each week on some form of mono-diet. This is a very individual thing – all people respond differently, and eating only apples or pears on one day each week might fit brilliantly into one person's schedule, yet be impossible for another's.

A simple diet of brown rice, steamed vegetables and lots of salad gives the body a wonderful rest and allows much background maintenance and healing work to be done. Following this for three days at a time will serve as a rejuvenating fillip for the whole system. If done during the summer months, more emphasis can be placed on the salad part of the meal, indeed you may wish to eat only raw food. In the winter, the addition of some cayenne pepper and ginger will help to keep the body warm.

Food combining is another tool that suits some people. Separating protein from carbohydrates can make things simpler on the digestion, and this can be done in a small way by eating the protein part of any meal first, the carbo-hydrate at the end. (In this scheme of food combining, vegetables with the exception of potatoes are considered neutral.) Others need to separate protein meals from carbohydrate meals altogether.

There are different types of fast – from a dry fast in which no food or drink is taken at all, to a mono-diet in which only one type of food is eaten. Dry fasting should never be attempted without the advice and monitoring of an experienced practitioner, but a day each week spent eating only apples, or pears, or drinking freshly made vegetable or fruit juices can be highly beneficial. It is in-advisable to follow a strict cleansing diet for more than three days without professional advice.

When detoxifying or following a mono-diet for a day or longer, it is important to keep warm and remember to drink lots of fresh, clean water. Any amount of exercise you do will reinforce the work of the diet and help liber-ate toxins. Energy levels may fluctuate, however, and it is common to feel lighter and more energetic, but not to have the usual amount of staying power – people often find they tire more easily. Sleep patterns may also alter – people usually find they need less sleep and wake feeling fresher, but may need to rest more than usual. All of this is because the extra energy liberated by making digestion less of a task is being used internally to mobilize the body's defences, pep-up the metabolism and, of course, to elimi-nate toxins.

Some of the first benefits to become obvious are a clear skin, which can be seen to almost glow; a brightness around the eyes, and a feeling of lightness which translates into the way we move – often noticed as a spring in the step, or a more confident posture. On longer-term diets (three days or more), the speed at which the body mobilizes toxins can for a time supersede the capability of the eliminative routes. This can lead to a period of experiencing mild headaches, some spots on the skin (particularly on the face) and feelings of lethargy. This never lasts for more than a day, and can be so mild as to pass almost unnoticed; it all depends on the individual level of health and vitality.

Most of these measures can be undertaken individually, but if assistance or support is required, your naturopath should be able to monitor your progress and make individual suggestions. Fasting and detoxifying are an important part of the naturopathic system of healthcare. Biologically, we are still hunter-gatherers; our systems are used to periods of fasting or low food intake, and eating large amounts of food *every* day is a relatively new idea. Regular detoxification allows our bodies time for rest and renewal within our busy schedules, and is a positive aid to preventative healthcare.

During the warmer months, spending a few days eating only raw food is an excellent way to boost the body's eliminative powers. During winter, the addition of cooked brown rice and steamed vegetables makes for a good clear out (in the colder weather you need the warmth from the cooked food). These mini-diets can be repeated once a month or, for a more sustained effect, spend one day each week on some form of fast.

Use the opportunity of following a detox diet to have a mental and emotional clear out too. Take the time to review your psychological and emotional well-being, and get rid of any dead wood. Make a list of those things that work in your life, and those that do not – and see how you can set about fixing or letting go of any aspects of your life, situations, or relationships that no longer serve you. Explore other ways of clearing out your life; the oriental art of Feng Shui suggests that clutter in the home can have a negative effect on health, so this may be the opportunity for a spring clean. Letting go of things you no longer need allows new energy to come in to your life, encourage this by making some time to appreciate beauty, experience the joys of nature, and become clearer about what you want to let in.

A Three-Day Detox Plan

- eating regular meals, even if they are small ones, is very important, so make sure that you have breakfast each day, and do not be tempted to skip any meal.
- make sure that you have some variety in your food – getting bored is one of the most common reasons for quitting any detox programme, so do not give yourself this excuse.
- drink lots and lots of good, clean water. Take a glass whenever you remember, and in the cold weather, drink it warm or hot.
- the foods you choose for your detox will depend on your own likes and dislikes, and what is seasonally available.

• do experiment a little by choosing new fruits and vegetables, and finding new combinations for them.

During these three days you will be choosing from:

all vegetables, with the exception of tomatoes, potatoes and spinach;

all fruits, with the exception of avocado pears, rhubarb, bananas and oranges;

all herbs with the exception of sorrel; (use these liberally to flavour meals and for their delicious taste).

You will also be adding a selection of the following spices and botanicals to your meals:

ginger, cinnamon, cloves, coriander leaf, garlic, black pepper (in moderation), cayenne pepper, cumin, turmeric and cardamon.

Use these to add warmth to meals, sprinkle on salads, use when cooking soup, etc. Garlic and ginger should form a part of every meal.

Have at least one portion of plain cooked short-grain brown rice every day.

Follow this detox for three days, and only do it once in every month. You should experience renewed energy levels during the first day, and after the third day, will notice a number of changes in your general health. Make sure that you break the diet well, having a gentle breakfast on Day Four, and avoiding any excesses for the next day or two.

Essentially, the more raw food you eat, the faster and more efficient the detox will be. However, it is important not to chill your digestive system, particularly during the cold weather, so a higher proportion of cooked food is eaten during the winter months. Then, the fact that you are eating a large amount of whole-grain rice does the work of cleaning your bowel, and the repetitive nature of the meals (e.g. only soup, or steamed vegetables) allows your digestive system to relax.

How you plan your detox will depend on the time of year – during the summer months you would have a medley of fruits or a fruit salad for breakfast, a large mixed salad and rice for lunch, and the same meal at dinner time.

During the winter, you need to keep your body warmer, so breakfast would be a savoury meal of steamed vegetables with rice, or even some vegetable broth. Lunch would be another warm meal of soup or steamed vegetables with rice, and dinner the same. Stewed fruit can be taken as a snack.

Vary the fruits and vegetables that you eat, and consider trawling the greengrocer's or supermarket shelf, and buying just one, or a small handful of everything that you see. Snack if you want to on fresh fruit and vegetables during the warmer months, and on vegetable broth during the winter.

Finding out more
Incorporated Society of British Naturopaths
Kingston
The Coach House
293 Gilmerton Road
Edinburgh EH16 5UQ
Tel: 0131 664 3435

Further Reading

Belinda Grant, *The Detox Diet Book*, Warner
Doris Grant and Jean Joice, *Food Combining for Health*, Thorsons
Henry Lindlahr, *Natural Therapeutics*, C. W. Daniel.

EXERCISE

Walking • Weight Training • Aquarobics

Exercise works the most important muscle in the body – the heart. As we work individual muscles or muscle groups, we improve the heart's capacity and ability to pump. This improved blood supply enables the muscles to work well and to grow, and general circulation is also improved. Although blood is pumped around the body, the lymphatic system (a fundamental part of our immune response and necessary for the removal of toxins) depends upon the mechanical effects of movement.

In order to strengthen the heart muscle, improve lung function, pep-up the circulation and the lymphatic system in this way, 20 minutes' exercise three times a week is necessary. To begin with, five minutes every day, or six days out of seven, is a good introduction, and will establish some form of exercise as a regular part of your daily routine. This also begins to stretch your body's capacity for exercise, and to prepare you for increased work as your fitness improves. This ability increases very quickly. The effects of sustained and regular exercise are amazing: within days stamina, strength and suppleness are increasing. It's almost as if these muscles have all been waiting and are ready to be stretched and tested, their response is so rapid.

For some, exercise is seen as a chore, and the only way to transform this into the life-enhancing event it should be is to find an enjoyable, interesting way to work out. The options are legion – if you enjoy nature, brisk walks may be the perfect way to begin any fitness campaign. **Walking** is an excellent all-round exercise that can improve muscle tone throughout the body; even peristalsis (the way food is moved through the gut) can be improved by regular walks. The abdominal muscles are gently squeezed and stretched with every step, and walking up hill is the most effective exercise for toning this area and it also makes the leg muscles work even harder. Wherever possible, walking on grass gives the best results, because it yields a little when you put your weight down, and sand has a similar quality.

Walking, and indeed all weight-bearing exercises, can be an important aid to women. Osteoporosis is a condition that can affect post-menopausal women – it causes the bones to become thinner and more brittle, so they fracture more easily. Regular weight-bearing exercise before, during and after the menopause has been shown to reduce the risk of suffering in this way.

Many people find that it is the social content of any activity that they enjoy the most. There are many contact sports that absolute beginners can join in with – they aren't all designed for professionals. Most small towns, community centres and even some firms have their own football, netball, rugby or rounders teams. Joining a sports and social club is a good idea in smaller communities, and most gyms will at least have a snack or juice bar where people can meet. The advantages of joining a centre like this range from club tournaments, which pit whichever members choose to sign on against each other, to the spontaneous situations which often arise when someone needs a partner for tennis, or an opponent for squash.

If time is an important consideration, there are many exercises that can be done at home. An exercise bike in front of an open window, or a bouncer (mini-trampoline) can provide a good aerobic workout at any point during the day. There is also an enormous range of exercise videos available that cover a wide variety of approaches – from Callanetics to cardiac funk. If you like dancing, then there are always discos and clubs to go to, or for a more social element there is a range of classes from jive and jazz to traditional Irish dancing. Exercise doesn't have to be all about sweaty bodies in bare-walled gymnasia; and you don't have to hurt to get fit.

If you would prefer a solitary pursuit, however, **weight training** is *all* about sweaty bodies in gyms. This form of workout is one of the most richly and immediately rewarding exercises I know of – after only a few weeks of body building you can see obvious visible changes in the size and shape of your whole body. After only a few sessions you can start to feel the difference. Initially this requires a strong commitment to visiting a gym four times a week for workouts, but very soon it can become positively addictive.

The natural pain-killers produced by the body, along with their mood-changing effects, and the fact that appetite is suppressed for a few hours after each workout, result in incredible 'highs'. These are the same feelings experienced by long-distance runners, joggers, and all athletes who work their bodies continuously. These feelings must contribute to the easy, swinging gait, bounce in the step and proud posture of all those who exercise regularly. Weight training is a perfect exercise form, and in combination with some form of weight-bearing exercise such as walking, running, or playing tennis, provides an all-round answer to women's health needs in their middle years.

Aquarobics is a very popular pursuit – a full-body aerobic workout in water. The benefits of this are enormous – working the body against the resistance of the water tones muscles much more quickly than any land-based exercise except weight training. It is gentle on the body, and enables the toning of specific areas without the punishing effects on the joints of conventional high-impact aerobics. And it incorporates all of the fun of messing about in the water.

During a class, the full range of exercises is clearly called out and exhibited by the teacher on the side of the pool, and the group in the water follow the teacher's lead. Most of the exercises are performed to music, and because they are performed in the shallow end with the group standing up or holding on to the side of the pool, non-swimmers can join in too. (Non-swimmers should tell the teacher, and may feel more comfortable staying close to the steps for the first few classes.)

The body is so well supported during water workouts that care must be taken not to overdo the amount of exercise taken initially, and also to execute the individual movements carefully, as the early signs of muscle tiredness and strain are not so obvious. Information on aquarobic classes can be obtained from most local authority swimming pools and sports centres.

After each class, there is often time set aside for the participants to swim. This ideal exercise for the whole body makes for a lovely finale to an exercise class and, once again, allows us the wonderful freedom of weightlessness and having fun in the element which supported us throughout our gestation. Spending time in the water is one of the only chances many of us get to relieve the pressures of gravity on our bodies and to experience the freedom that this can engender.

Whatever form of exercise you choose, it is important to ensure that you are properly equipped. This doesn't only apply to specialist pursuits like rock climbing or scuba diving – walkers need proper shoes that offer good support and tread, and a decent support bra; cyclists really need safety helmets and, if cycling through traffic, face masks to limit the amount of poisons inhaled. Weight trainers and others using any type of machinery or equipment must be properly trained in their use to ensure good results as well as from the safety point of view.

If you choose any activities that involve jumping – from high-impact aerobics to jogging, you must ensure the safety of the surface and wear good protective shoes with support. Well-sprung floors in dance studios and gyms do much to cushion the joints, but proper footwear is essential. (As is a decent support bra.) Jogging on grass is much safer, and a better exercise, than running on concrete or stone. Even with running shoes, the jarring effect on all the joints is just terrible. It is also worth bearing in mind that if you exercise in the open air, you are likely to be breathing in dangerous levels of pollution at a very fast rate (especially if you are in a town or city, and jogging anywhere near its centre, or along a busy road).

Every sport or exercise has its own guidelines and necessities, and finding out about these before you start can guard against any mishaps. All exercising requires a warm-up period, or some sort of preparatory movement. Usually these are gentle stretching and toning exercises, and they can form an enjoyable routine in their own right, especially if done to music or in the company of others. They can also be a good way to zero in on any specific body areas that need extra attention: the abdominal muscles, for example; and are excellent for improving suppleness generally.

Movement is a true sign of life – a positively identifiable sign that we are alive. Positively one of the best ways to maintain our 'aliveness' is through exercise. It maintains the mobility of our joints, helps regulate the metabolism, improves muscle tone and size, increases our oxygen capacity and improves posture. Exercise lets our bodies work more efficiently, so we feel better and look good. (See also Body Forms for a new slant on exercise.)

Finding out more
The Sports Council
Regional addresses for UK in the UK telephone directory.

FELDENKRAIS METHOD

This is a system of realignment in which the emphasis is on re-educating the body's postural muscles (see Alexander Technique, p. 18). It seeks to retrain the body through an awareness of, and sensitivity to, movement, which is encouraged through a system of gentle exercises. To take away the pressures of gravity, these are all initially practised with the client or student lying on the ground.

Moshe Feldenkrais was an atomic physicist, and had studied engineering. A knee injury led him to begin his investigations into the dynamics of human movement. A black belt in judo, he drew on his knowledge of martial arts to develop his method, which relates the mechanics of the body to patterns of learning and behaviour. He also worked with F.M. Alexander and explored yoga, psychology and spiritual philosophies. He maintained that by releasing negative physical patterns, restrictive mental patterns would also change.

The method is taught in two ways: awareness through movement is taught in groups, with a teacher leading the class through a range of simple movements. These may be everyday movements such as flexing the feet, or exercises that are designed to heighten the individual's awareness of the way they use their body. Asked to bend and lower one knee, for example, people may find that they tense a number of unrelated body parts, such as the hands, and even the face. Functional integration is the second part of the method. This takes place in individual sessions when the practitioner will interact with, and guide the student's body through the range of movements.

The movements are all very gentle and can be used by young and old alike. They have been shown to be particularly beneficial for people with special needs, and for people when in recovery. The key to the method is in the conscious awareness of movement, and the way this can effect beneficial mental and emotional, as well as physical, change.

The Feldenkrais Information Centre,
188 Old Street
London EC1V 9BP
Tel: 0181 584 8819

Further Reading

Moshe Feldenkrais, *Awareness through Movement*, Penguin.

FLOWER REMEDIES

The distilled essences of flowers can be used for their therapeutic effects on both the emotional and physical levels.

A retired English doctor, Edward Bach, first started to use flower essences, or remedies, at the turn of the century. He combined his knowledge of psychological typing and emotional states with his love of nature, and began to explore the therapeutic use of flowers. In his early morning walks, he collected the dew which had settled on the petals of an assortment of flowers, and explored their effects on his own emotions. Through time, he evolved a system of determining the effects of a number of different flowers, and set about making the remedies available commercially.

He experimented with letting the petals steep in water, and then exposing them to sunlight to allow the preparation to be infused with the healing qualities of the flowers. He later added alcohol as a preservative, to enable them to be bottled and, now, exported around the world.

His theory that different diseases were directly related to emotional types or temperaments led him to make seven classifications of personality, which are then subdivided to make a specific diagnosis easier. His definitions were oversensitivity, fear, uncertainty or indecision, lack of interest in the present, despondency and despair, over-concern for the welfare of others, and loneliness.

Oversensitivity, for example, has four different remedies – agrimony for anxiety and mental torment hidden by a brave face; centaury for a weak will or co-dependent habits; walnut for major life changes and holly for jealousy and suspicion.

Perhaps his best known combination of flower essences is Rescue Remedy – a mix of five different remedies: cherry plum, clematis, impatiens, rock rose and star of Bethlehem. This was designed as the perfect first-aid measure for shock and anxiety. To quote Bach's own writings, 'It is an all purpose composite for effects of anguish, examinations, going to the dentist, etc. Comforting, calming and reassuring to those distressed by startling experiences.' Its use, though, is restricted to non-medical emergencies because of the alcohol content of the mixture, although it can be used externally in such instances, and has been proven to be extremely effective when used in this way.

Since this pioneering work, the use of flower essences has developed further, and now there are remedies that incorporate both earth and sea flowers from different parts of the world. The many varieties now available are known as Flower Essences, marking them as distinct from the Bach Flower Remedies, and there are full ranges from Hawaii, a variety from the USA and Canada, also from India, Australia and New Zealand, Africa and the Amazon, as well as other varieties from Britain and elsewhere in Europe.

Some of these remedies are potentized in different ways, or contain vodka instead of brandy, or in some cases no alcohol at all. Andreas Korte Essences from the Amazon are among those that do not even damage the flowers – they use a crystal filled with natural spring water to capture the essence of the flower, leaving it growing and alive.

The Australian Bush Essences and the Living Essences of Australia draw on the ancient knowledge of the indigenous Aboriginal people, who have been using flowers to heal themselves for over 10,000 years. By contrast, some of the flower remedies have been developed very recently. Desert Alchemy Flower Essences were born of an inspirational experience in 1983, when Cynthia Athina Kemp was driving through the Arizona Desert and was able to touch the extraordinary qualities of some of the Saguaro cacti, and other wild plants. This is all in sharp contrast to the Bach Flower Remedies, which are now made by machine.

The small 10 or 20ml bottles in which the remedies or essences are sold each contain a dropper, and the idea is to take two to three drops on the tongue, or in a small glass of water, which is then very slowly sipped.

With some remedies, particularly Rescue Remedy, the effect can be felt immediately, although they all have a long-term effect too. Those working on depression, chronic situations or deep-seated feelings can all be taken regularly – first thing in the morning, last thing at night, and two or three times during the day – to achieve the best results.

Many of the remedies can also be taken for the fleeting

moods of everyday life. The simplest way to do this is to mix a little of the remedy or remedies of your choice with some spring water and keep them in a small dropper bottle – these can be bought at any pharmacy.

The remedies can be used externally too – a few drops of elm added to hot water in which a compress is then soaked can provide tremendous ease for strained or pulled ligaments when applied to the area. Crab apple can be added to a cold water wash for boils or bad spots, and Rescue Remedy applied to a bruise speeds up recovery. Its use in this way became so popular that there is now available a lanolin-free rescue remedy cream. The drops or the cream make an excellent first-aid remedy for minor burns; apply a little cream to the burn, and take one drop on the tongue to promote a total speedy recovery.

The remedies can be used by children, again bearing in mind the alcohol content, as an excellent first-aid remedy for the trauma of minor accidents. They are also said to be quite effective for treating animals, and also plants. A few drops of rescue remedy added to the water for a distressed plant should soon pep it up.

A list of the full range of flower remedies can be obtained wherever the remedies are sold, and each essence is itemized alongside a few key words to enable self-diagnosis. Many counsellors and therapists use flower remedies alongside their work. These can help ease or resolve painful feelings as they come up.

The remedies can be taken at any time, and there are no contra-indications, or side effects, to their use, except that they contain alcohol, which may prohibit their use by some people. Because you only take a small amount at a time –

usually just a few drops – the alcohol content should not stop you driving or fulfilling any other obligations.

Dr Bach also worked as a homeopath, and as such was used to dealing with the subtler aspects of medicine. He was content to state that the healing energy of the flowers transferred itself to the water solution in which they were soaked. Having a small bottle of the remedy was, obviously, easier than having to find the flower itself, particularly for those not living in the countryside or without the knowledge to correctly identify each plant. The bottling remedies also meant that each remedy would be available throughout the year, not just when the flower itself was in bloom.

Today we eat the flowers, leaves, stems and roots of plants for their nutritious and health-giving qualities, and bathe in the fragrance of their essential oils, so it is only a small step to accepting that the water in which flower petals sit in the preparation of each remedy can easily absorb the potent qualities of flowers.

I keep some remedies close to hand – my own favourites: Rescue Remedy for trauma; crab apple for its cleansing qualities; rock rose for fear and terror (terrific for stage fright!); and olive for fatigue. People soon find their own favourites, and those which help at different times.

Flower remedies and some essences are available at many health food shops, chemists and natural health clinics. The full current listing of Flower Essence families is growing all the time, and this list shows those that are available in the UK, with their country of origin.

Andreas Korte Essences (Africa and the Amazon)
Bush Flower Essences (Australia)
Living Essences of Australia
New Perception Flower Essences (New Zealand)
Bailey Essences (UK)
Findhorn Flower Essences (Scotland)
Green Man Tree Essences (UK)
Harebell Remedies (UK)
Deva Flower Elixirs (France)
Himalayan Aditi, Himalayan Flower Enhancers, and Himalayan Indian Tree and Flower Essences (India)
Alaskan Flower and Environmental Essences
Desert Alchemy Flower Essences (Arizona, USA)
FES and California Research Essences, Flower Essence Society, and Master's Flower Essences (California, USA)
Pegasus Essences (Colorado, USA)
Hawaiian Tropical Flower Essences
Petite Fleur Essences, and Perelandra Virginian Rose and Garden Essences (Texas, USA)
Pacific Essences and Flower and Gem Remedy Association (Canada)

Do not be daunted by the extent of available remedies – let it reassure you that whatever your concerns there is undoubtedly already at least one remedy especially for it. Let your intuition guide you, and explore whatever ranges you feel drawn to. Check the information on them for the things that matter to you – you may, for example, choose to avoid those with alcohol, or those whose origins you do not know.

Once you feel drawn to a particular remedy you can take it directly on your tongue, or add it to a small glass of water. You may wish to take a combination of different remedies at any one time, and this is possible even if they come from different sources or countries. You can choose the remedies and make them up into a mother remedy, in one of two ways, which you will continue to take for a period of time, perhaps one month.

1. For this you will need a large dropper bottle (available from your chemist) which you have rinsed through with spring water. Choose the remedies that you are going to be taking, and put four drops of each one into a large bottle. Add one teaspoon of brandy or vodka (depending on what is used in the individual remedies), and top up to the brim with spring water. If you do not wish to use alcohol, add clear honey instead. Label this clearly with the combination details, and the date.

You may also like to note what the mix is for, as well as the flower essences it contains. Use this mother recipe every day just as you would a single remedy, taking a few drops directly on your tongue, or adding to a small glass of water. Take the remedy about five times each day, especially first thing in the morning, and last thing at night. You may like to keep a record of your responses and the changes that occur in relation to the issues for which you chose these remedies. Continue through the month, and then take a week's rest, before deciding whether to carry on taking this mixture, or perhaps choose another, or even to not take any.

2. The other useful way to take a mixture of remedies is to add two drops of each to a small bottle of spring water, which you can keep in the fridge. This will keep for a maximum of

---

five days, and is an excellent way to take the remedies easily
and without anybody else noticing – you can carry the bottle
out with you if necessary, and these days taking a sip from a
bottle of mineral water is not the least bit unusual. I recommend
this if you plan to only take the remedies for a short time, or if
you plan to choose new combinations every few days. Once
again, you can sip some of the water, or pour it into a glass,
and take some about five times during the day, especially first
thing in the morning and last thing at night.

Finding out more
The Edward Bach Centre
Mount Vernon
Sotwell
Wallingford
Oxon OX10 0PZ
Tel: 01491 39489 or 34678
Flower Essence Society
P O Box 459
Nevada City
California 95959
Tel: (800) 548 0075 or (916) 265 0258

Further Reading

Edward Bach, *Heal Thyself*, C.W. Daniel Company
Clare G. Harvey with Amanda Cochrane, *The Encyclo-
paedia of Flower Remedies*, Thorsons.

GROUP WORK

Encounter Groups • Therapy Groups • Family Groups
• Assertiveness Training • Family Therapy

There must be nearly as many reasons for joining a group as there are different groups to join! In the main, the reasons can be divided into three broad categories: to learn a particular skill or set of skills, e.g. assertiveness training; to seek to resolve a particular situation that involves others, e.g. family therapy; to share experiences and a support network, e.g. growth groups. Being in a group can, in part, satisfy our basic human need for contact and social interaction. This is something that is very important to us, and it is often missing from our modern lives. The loss of the extended family and increasing industrialization can make us feel alone, isolated and alienated. Joining with a group of some sort is a good idea, if only to remind us of our shared purpose. It has wonderful healing spin-offs, too, e.g. eating a meal with friends; good company can benefit you more than eating alone.

The structure and regularity of group meetings will vary – sometimes a leader, facilitator or trainer will provide a focus for the group, or the organization and input will be shared by all. Most often a commitment is required as far as attendance is concerned, although some groups are far more informal, operating on an 'as needed' or drop-in basis. This is most often the case with support organizations such as Alcoholics Anonymous and Narcotics Anonymous.

The women's consciousness-raising groups I went to in the 1970s used a completely open structure – with people committing to one meeting at a time, no chair person, and the venue alternating among the homes of the members. This apparent lack of formal structure encouraged the personal responsibility and individual contribution of all involved.

Obviously the structure and agenda of any group will, to a large degree, be determined by its cause – why the group has formed; but there are many common factors. In groups we may learn more about the way we relate to others, how those interactions affect us, and how we are perceived by others. The inevitable exchange of views, opinions and feelings can lead to improved social skills and a greater self-knowledge, whether or not these are direct aims.

The support and understanding offered by a group can build confidence and create a secure forum in which to express one's deeper feelings. If membership is mixed in terms of age, gender, interests, social background, etc., then the group can become a microcosm of society, providing us with a sample of reality in which new stances and forms of expression can be explored. More defined groups; those with a particular purpose or specific membership, can provide a unique opportunity for solidarity.

The prospect of joining a group can be daunting for some – conjuring up embarrassing memories of school-time pressures to 'contribute'. The warm, supportive nature of most groups, however, soon puts people at their ease. Most often, there is no pressure to speak or participate actively, although some groups begin by going round and giving everybody the opportunity to introduce themselves, often just by saying their name.

Of course not all groups are growth-related – nor do they need to be able to provide the benefits of working closely with others. If the purpose is to make social contacts and interact with others, a host of activity-based groups is available – from formalized role playing as in amateur dramatic societies, to re-enactment situations like the Tolkien society (they gather and act out situations from his books; often meeting over weekends and setting up living and social conditions to fit each theme). These could be seen as the ultimate in play therapy!

Gatherings of any people who share a common interest whether it be archery, a health condition, or a life purpose, provide a valuable opportunity to understand more about ourselves and how we function in society. As a rule, most people gain from joining with others in this way in direct proportion to their openness to new ideas, and the generosity with which they share their own experiences.

To name just a few, there are **encounter groups, therapy groups, family groups**, those that meet to discuss dream analysis, to meditate, to learn the physical expression of their feelings, and for mutual support. Information about local and national groups can be found in libraries, citizens advice bureaux and adult education centres.

Common to all growth-related groups is the sense of making a safe and confidential place where support, or whatever else is needed, can be given and received. It can be very reassuring to hear one's own fears or anxieties being voiced by other people; and this can help us all gain some perspective on our own discomfort. For those without any particular worries, groups can often provide the opportunity to refine their skill in establishing relationships. They can also give us the chance to give of ourselves or our experience in a relaxed setting.

In groups with a specific purpose, **assertiveness training**, for example, all the group members will be involved in acting out potential situations and practising their responses. This can lead to real breakthroughs when the insights and actions of others can be focused to provide some truly effective strategies. Often, what may seem simple, or like a natural response to one person, can provide the perfect solution to a situation that seemed impossible to someone else. Acting out the situations also allows you to try things on for size – to see whether a particular solution suits your way of being, and whether behaving in a particular way lets you feel good about yourself in the company of other people.

Family therapy and other problem-solving endeavours benefit from the objectivity of the group facilitator, leader or therapist. To change familiar patterns of behaviour requires us first to notice them, and this is something for which we often need either distance or the observations of an onlooker to achieve. The old cliché of not seeing the wood for the trees is most pertinent when applied to relationships, because we are involved so intimately that we often cannot gain the perspective that allows us to see things from an objective position. Although this works most effectively when all family members or involved parties are present within the group, much headway can be made with only some. This also works well for partnership difficulties.

Loneliness is a growing problem in our society. The more complex, industrialized and urban our living conditions, the more isolation people are inclined to feel. With the breakdown of local communities and ever smaller family units, our need for company becomes greater. The real gift of group situations is in the opportunity they provide for people to truly meet – to share what is important to them as individuals while leaving behind a lot of the labels – to step out of any constraining roles they must play in their everyday lives and be themselves.

Finding out more

Alcoholics Anonymous
11 Radcliffe Gardens
London SW10
Tel: 0181 352 3001

Family Therapy
Association of Ireland
17 Dame Court
Dublin 2
Tel: 01 679 4055

Institute for Dream Analysis
1 Daleham Gardens
London NW3 5BY
Tel: 0171 431 2693

Institute of Family Therapy
43 New Cavendish Street
London W1
Tel: 0171 935 1651

HEALING

Healing is, in a sense, what all of this book is concerned with – uniting mind, body and spirit in a balanced, health-giving way.

There are many forms of healing; sometimes it takes place between mother and child, or between lovers, or friends who really care about each other. This is a natural, human thing, and it can happen when we need it to. Healing is also a personal process, and we heal ourselves as well and as early as we can. We may seek help from others on occasion, or encounter it, but any personal transformation is by its very nature a very individual thing.

Healers help others by providing the energy that is needed for the patient or client to heal themselves. This may take the form of physical work, or emotional support, or counselling; the important thing is not so much how it is offered, but the way in which it is received. As self-righting organisms we take what we need in order to facilitate our own healing.

Some healers call themselves faith healers, or spiritualist healers. For some faith healers, the fact that they believe it works is enough; others require the person receiving the healing to have faith in them. There is an important distinction between spiritual healers, who maintain that their work is spiritual in its nature, and Spiritualist healers who have their own church and organized religious beliefs.

Many healers simply call themselves healers, or psychic or natural healers. All healing is natural. Most psychic healers place an emphasis on the counselling aspect of any work they do, believing that conscious awareness of the nature of any difficulty – how it arose, what compounds it, etc., is an integral part of any healing process. There is no point in repairing something if you don't know how it got upset in the first place. Without such knowledge, there is every possibility of it occurring again. Shamans, Wise Women, and other true healers all work with the patient or client, involving them in as direct a way as possible to aid their understanding of their situation.

Although many of the lessons that we need to learn in life may have to be repeated, we can avoid a lot of problems by completing things properly. This means being able to respond and react to what is happening right now, and taking the right action in order to ensure that we leave no loose ends. This can also lead us to reach back into the past to find the cause of any complaint. Psychics, Shamans, and other healers can aid such journeys, and also help by discovering the level of any disorder – its root may be physical and affected by diet, for example, or it may be emotional, or energetic. Some of our problems can be caused, or at least compounded, by a lack of understanding. This is where suitable counselling can work to bring other matters to our attention and alter our level of awareness.

What happens in a healing session will vary according to the type of healer. Most often they involve 'hands-on' work, when the healer will gently touch the body at a variety of sites. Sometimes healers work using other techniques – they may have studied some form of healthcare; perhaps physically based like cranio-sacral therapy, or maybe more system-related like herbalism. They can then combine their knowledge with the healing ability to achieve the best possible outcome.

When using hands-on work, the healer may use both their hands to 'sandwich' particular parts of the body, or they may be placed some distance apart. People describe the feelings as being warming, or tingling; some find a refreshing coolness under the healer's hands, and memories or thoughts may come into the mind. Sometimes people see images, or colours weaving themselves around the healer and themselves. Each experience is different – those needing to find peace usually feel calm and restful; a depressed individual may feel pleasantly energized after a session. Some people may not be aware of any sensations at all, but feel somewhat different, or changed afterwards.

This work can also be done without touching the patient or client. Healers work mainly by interacting with a person's energetic state, and this extends beyond the body to form the aura. Some psychics can see this, others feel it or sense it, and many find they prefer to work in this way. This may involve the healer holding or moving their hands off the body, but close to its surface. Sometimes, they can be some distance away. Once again, the person receiving the healing may be aware of changes in temperature or a variety of sensations, including emotional releases during the session. Usually these take place with the person seated, but they can be lying down, on a treatment couch, or even standing.

A person's energy constellates around, or can be seen to emanate from, a number of centres around the body. In the East these are known as chakras (wheels of energy), and the major ones lie along the mid-line of the body, extending from the top of the head down to the feet. Each centre relates to a different drive or motivational energy, e.g. courage, creativity, inspiration, etc. These centres, being comprised of energy, also have a colour, a sound or harmonic, a texture, etc. Colours are easiest to see, and many psychics and other healers see or sense them and use this information to assess a person's overall health. A grass-green relates to the creativity centre; yellow corresponds to the solar or courage centre; pink to the emotional and physical energy from the heart centre; mauve to the communication centre in the throat; and blue to the centre for motivation and inspiration. Other healing systems use other ways to interpret what is happening with the person.

Quartz crystals can help encourage, support and re-balance the energy centres; rose quartz is good for the heart centre, and can balance emotion, and sapphire can clear the inspiration centre in the head. These are sometimes used during a session, or you may see one on the healer's desk. Quartz crystal works like a battery, and the energy from the healer can connect with the energy of the crystal to be transferred to the client. Psychics may also wear a crystal or a gemstone to balance their own energies, and they may also be used as a pendulum to aid diagnosis and answer other queries. Individual crystals have their own energy, like all living things, and some are more suited to working with people, or for use in healing. It is important to choose and care for these companions with respect for their own uniquenes.

Some healers use coloured lights to impress the consciousness of the client, some even use little black boxes and don't call themselves healers at all.

Healing energy can also be transmitted over long distances – the person can be miles away or in another country. Many healers keep absent or distant healing lists, and they will send healing energy to people who are experiencing difficulties but who cannot see them in person.

Some people believe that the ability to heal is a gift, and as such it must be freely shared. These people either work for nothing, or ask for a donation. Most professional healers, like all other practitioners, charge for their sessions. They realize that we have to give and receive, and find balance in this as in all other actions and activities. Appointments usually last between thirty minutes and one hour, although timings do vary.

There are no associations that cover the whole profession, mainly because of the wide range of different techniques used by healers. Individual knowledge, interpretation skills and beliefs vary as enormously in this profession as does expertise. Personal referral is really the only way to find a healer, or you could decide to approach the spiritualist church.

Your body is healing itself as you read this – it works all the time to keep you as well as it can. It is your physical home throughout your visit here on earth, and makes every effort to ensure that it is as useful as it can be. Healing can work in an instant, and you will probably have experienced this for yourself, in the reassuring hug from a friend, or a caring comment from another. The following exercise is a powerful way to augment your own healing ability, and it will form a useful aid that you can use anywhere, and anytime. This is always a favourite exercise in my classes, and one that students say is most useful to them.

The healing palette

Sit or lie down in a comfortable position, and take a few deep, relaxed breaths. Feel yourself to be centred and calm, and imagine any tensions leaving your body every time you breathe out. Know that you are safe, and secure in your own energy, and that any worries or concerns will not trouble you now. Continue your deep, restful breathing for a few minutes, establishing a nice comforting rhythm.

1. Close your eyes, if they are not already shut, and clear the view that you see in front of you. Let any images you see settle and leave you with a thick, dark expanse that is rich with texture, yet completely blank. Imagine it as a pair of thick dark velvet curtains that have been drawn across a stage shutting out all light, or use whatever other scene inspires you. Keep your breathing deep, calm, and rhythmic, and do not allow any physical tensions or awareness to interrupt your imaging.

2. Slowly, and one at a time, start to see some light forming on the surface of your darkness. Tiny specks at first, that now slowly come together to begin to form something that you

can recognize. As these minute pieces of light move towards each other, become aware that they are uniting to form a sea of swirling colours – muted and pastel or distant at first, and gently becoming more solid and brighter. Notice the green that is tending to settle towards the bottom of this grouping, and appreciate its particular shade. Next you will see the clear and vibrant yellow that rests above it, reminding you of a golden sun on a wonderful warm day. See how these two colours interact with each other, gently touching and moving together in a wonderful dance of light.

Look above them and you will be able to discern a strikingly beautiful pink that is shot through with different shades of itself. Feel the warmth of this colour, and notice the harmony between all the colours that you now see. Becoming clearer now, above the pink is a delicate mauve. It may be hard to pull yourself away from the stunning pink, but it's all right because it will stay there and you will still be able to see it, but now the subtler, delicate mauve is attracting your attention – look straight at it, and see the elegant colour shifts between it and the pink. Rising now, the mauve shimmers and changes, and above it you see a clear blue, that becomes clearer as you look at it.

3. All your colours have stabilized now, and you can see them as you look down: the clear blue is closest to you, then it segues into a gentle mauve that rises up from that stunning pink. This sits atop your strong yellow, and your vibrant green. See them all as they are, beautiful and different – quite distinct, yet all having come from the same source. Really look at your colours, so that you will remember your own distinctive shades and hues, and commit them to memory.

4. Notice now which colour in particular twinkles at you or calls your attention. Take your time and see if this happens. If so, go to it and simply bask in the centre of that colour, stabilizing it with your presence, and bathing in its light. If no colour beckons, take your time and enjoy the sight of all of them in their harmony in front of you. Remember to keep breathing, and allow the gentle rhythm of your breaths to hold you in this place.

You are seeing your own palette of colours, and this is a wonderful thing. If any of them is not as clear as the others, or does not appear in the same place as I have described, that is fine, just enjoy whatever colour show you are seeing, and do not worry.

5. Take your time, and when you are ready take a big deep breath, and as you breathe out, see the colours before you stream up into the air above you, and form above your head. Let them stay there for just an instant, before falling down all around you in a fantastic shower of coloured light. Bathe in this light/colour shower for as long as you like, feeling your body become refreshed and energized as the colours fall around you, and as you reabsorb all that you need in through your skin. See the colour intensity lessen, as more and more of the coloured light is accepted back inside your body, and feel the tremendous sense of warmth and well-being that this brings.

6. Slowly, the colour will lessen until it almost disappears. Keep your eyes closed for a moment longer, and then take another big, deep breath in, and as you breathe out, open your eyes. Rest for a few minutes and revel in the feelings and sights that you have just experienced. You can return to this

exercise any time you choose, and now you know your current colour spectrum, you may choose to include some of these in your life – in the clothes you wear, your furnishing and decorations, and in the places you like to be.

Most people can sense physical energy quite easily. This exercise will hone those skills for you, and may even convince you, if you were in any doubt. Practise this with a friend, partner or family member, and be prepared for a whole new world of discovery.

1. Rub your hands together vigorously, and shake your shoulders to relieve any tension there. You might like to turn to the section on shiatsu (pp. 278–84) and spend a few minutes doing some Do-in to wake up your body. Take a few deep breaths, and close your eyes to get a sense of how you are feeling right now. Be aware of your body and your energy, and how comfortable you are feeling. When you open your eyes, be ready to experience something new.

2. Ask your friend to sit down on the floor, or on an upright chair, with space around them for you to move freely. Tell them that you are going to gently sense their energy (afterwards you can change places). Stand at a right angle to your friend (or kneel if they are sitting on the floor), and rub your hands together again until they tingle, and you feel alert and energized. Hold them up about ten inches above your friend's head, and about three feet apart. You are going to slowly bring them down, one in front and one behind your friend's body, keeping them off the surface of their skin, and without

touching them. Close your eyes, and be aware of looking at your friend through the eyes in the palms of your hands.

3. It may take a few minutes for you to switch to seeing in this way, but that is fine, just take your time. Lower your hands exquisitely slowly, until you sense that you are closer to them. Do not be tempted to open your eyes, trust your hands. This is not any kind of race to get your hands to reach the floor, it is an amazing opportunity to begin to see some of the beauty of our existence.

4. You are going to gently scan with your hands and the whole of your awareness, until your hands come down to the floor. You may sense areas where you feel you want to stay, or that you want to move quickly past; or some spots may feel cool, like there is a gentle breeze blowing there; or you may perceive yourself as being close to a heat source. Perhaps thoughts or images come to mind when you are in a particular spot, or you sense a feeling or emotion. Everyone perceives things differently, so any or all of these is possible, and you may find other ways of your own to express what you are sensing. If you feel like lingering in a spot, linger there for as long as you feel you want to. If somewhere makes you feel like hurrying on, do so. Follow the signs and information that you are given, and trust it.

5. When you have finally finished, and your hands have reached the floor, take a moment for yourself before opening your eyes and sharing your experience with your friend. Just take a few deep breaths, and return to the sense of yourself that you had at the start of this exercise. Take a moment to review for yourself what you have experienced, and how you feel now.

6. When you are quite ready, share your story with your friend. Often they will have had some awareness of your hands, and may have their own experiences to share with you. It sometimes comes as a surprise when people's feelings and sensings are grounded in this reality – like feeling heat over the site of a newly digested dinner, or over the rapidly healing site of a recently broken bone. Sometimes colours, temperature changes and strong emotions are felt, at other times the sensations can be as subtle as a whisper. Share all of this with your friend, because it is theirs, and repeat the experience whenever you like. It will be different with other people, when you are feeling different, and it will change as you become more experienced at working in this way.

Further Reading

Betty Balcombe, *As I See It*, Piatkus
Michael Harner, *The Way of the Shaman*, HarperCollins
Gerald Jampoulski, *Love is Letting Go of Fear*, Foundation for Inner Peace
W. Brugh Joy, *Joy's Way*, J.P. Tarcher Inc.

HERBS

The use of herbs and plants for their nutritional and curative properties is a well-documented part of our history. Herbs were our earliest form of medicine. Their nutritional benefits and healing powers have been known for centuries. From the papyrus documents of Ancient Egypt, and the earliest Chinese writings come detailed records of the uses and values of a variety of plants and herbs, many of which are still used today. Many of the herbs now commonly used in Europe travelled from the Mediterranean, courtesy of the Egyptians and the Romans, but each continent has its own indigenous plants.

Nowadays, our laboratories are busy distilling the active properties of plants for use in the pharmaceutical industry as though it were only this part that was important. Much of the medication currently available is copied or extracted from nature: digitalis, a powerful heart drug, from foxgloves; quinine from the bark of the cinchona tree; cancer-inhibiting drugs from tropical plants; pain-killers from poppies; and aspirin from the willow tree. Some 25 per cent of modern medicines are synthetic copies of the active principles in plants.

As medical science investigates further, so new

discoveries are made and then copied or synthesized, concentrated, and provided to the public in a form that bears little resemblance to the original natural remedy. In the main, the active constituents in plants are not locked away as some sort of pique on the part of nature, they are mixed with other substances which aid their absorption, make digestion easier, combat any potential side-effects, or make assimilation easier. If they are not available in large amounts, it is because a small dose is usually more effective.

Many naturopaths use herbs extensively, and there is a host of herbs that can be used in the home. In the main, these will be eaten fresh, or dried, and can be added to meals or drunk as infusions or teas. They can also be applied externally as compresses or poultices, or diluted to form valuable washes and added to baths.

Many modern herbalists or medical herbalists tend to work exclusively with herbs, although some will also use wider dietary measures. They will usually prescribe the herbs as tinctures or decoctions (liquids which are distillations of the herbs themselves mixed with alcohol). This means that they can be taken as a 'medicine' – one 5ml dose twice a day, for example – although this method makes it difficult for those with any alcohol intolerance and those who avoid alcohol altogether.

The old-school herbalist, however, will often have a much wider appreciation of the use and preparation of herbs, and their role in the diet. They are more likely to suggest other health-promoting measures, and have a keen knowledge of the need for proper diet, elimination and exercise to enhance the work of the herbs themselves. This is where you are likely to encounter a richness of remedies and a much wider variety of medicinal forms, including elixirs, cordials, boluses, syrups and tisanes.

Practitioners of Chinese herbal medicine use herbs grown in the Orient, within the framework of Oriental medicine. They diagnose according to traditional principles, assessing the nature of the individual, the disorder, and the chosen herbs and diet in terms of the energetic values, e.g. hot or cold, yin or yang, etc., (see p. 54)

Herbs have a toning effect on the tissues of the body, and are often able to restore function to disordered or imbalanced organs and systems. Individual herbs will have an affinity with a particular organ or system: parsley is a kidney tonic; dandelion a liver tonic; and red clover has a cleansing action on the lymphatic system. Some of the herb's efficacy can be attributed to its vitamin and mineral content, which will be easily taken up by the body. Nettles are particularly high in iron, and rose-hips are a good source of vitamin C.

Each herb or plant comprises a sometimes complicated group of properties, and this balance of active and inactive ingredients can aid absorption and prevent side-effects. (The majority of herbs have none, the few that do will be handled with care by a trained practitioner.) Side-effects do occur, however, when the active principles are isolated or concentrated, as in prescription drugs. Herbs have a rapid action in the body, and it is important to combine them correctly and monitor amount or dosage, and frequency, in order to gain their full benefit. Overdosage is rarely dangerous, again unlike the synthetic versions.

Psychics and some other people can have a high level of sensitivity or affinity with herbs as well as with other forms of medicine and treatment. By eating or taking herbs in their natural form, it is easy to control the amount and frequency of intake, and therefore the beneficial effects. As a general rule, the fresh herb will be most active and effective, although careful drying preserves many of the herb's properties and is the most suitable method for storage. Once dried, the herb needs to be protected from light and heat if it is not to deteriorate.

The use of herbs can be short-term and specific, or more general and ongoing. Fresh or dried yarrow may be taken as a tea several times a day to help with a case of cystitis, yet it may also be recommended as an ongoing support – a cup once or twice a week throughout the season to continue cleansing the area.

Although most herbs can be taken internally in this way, a number can be very effective when applied externally, and this may be one of the forms recommended by your practitioner. You may be prescribed herbs individually or in groups by your naturopath as part of their recommendations for ongoing healthcare. Visits to a herbalist will often begin with the taking of your health history, and the use of some other form of diagnosis to back up their decisions; many herbalists also use iridology for this purpose. The initial consultation will last anything up to an hour, and subsequent visits will vary from 20–30 minutes. The second visit will enable the herbalist to note your response to the herbs they have suggested, and it is most important to keep this appointment. Subsequent visits may continue for as long as the complaint lasts, or if constitutional work is being done, may be as often as once a month over a year or more.

The table below shows the home applications of some common herbs, many of which you may be used to adding to meals for their culinary properties. Herbs used in cooking often have a particular effect on digestion – caraway, cardamon and other seeds found in curried sauces prevent flatulence. The cloves that are so regularly added to winter meals are excellent for the circulation, and the nutmeg sprinkled on night-time drinks is a natural tranquilliser.

All of these herbs are safe to use as first-aid measures, although this form of prescription should never be substituted for a visit to a practitioner. If the measure is not effective, or the situation recurs, this could be a symptom of another complaint, so use these recommendations with discretion.

Care must always be taken during pregnancy, and herbs should not be taken without the advice and monitoring of your healthcare practitioner.

Herb	Home Uses
Calendula	This has extensive healing properties, particularly for skin, and in the treatment of fungal conditions. Use as a cream for cuts and grazes. Add to the bath or as a gargle for thrush. Take as a tea once a week for internal cleansing and healing
Chamomile	A calming, digestion-enhancing herb, with strong eliminative qualities. Soothing for the nervous system, take as a tea to relieve biliousness and flatulence. A good after-dinner drink. The cold tea makes a soothing eye-wash

Fennel	Soothing for the digestion, and useful to aid sore throats. This is a main constituent of gripe water, and can be taken as a weak tea to aid digestion. Good as a gargle too
lady's mantle	A 'women's' herb. Take as a tea to bring energy to the pelvis, help regulate periods and strengthen the womb. Can also be added to the bath water (as directions in text for Calendula)
Marjoram	This is sedative and relaxing. Take as a tea to relieve period pains, nervous headache and acid indigestion. Do not take more than one cup a day. To relieve the pain of colic, use as a pack by heating the dried herb and wrapping around the abdomen in a tea-towel or strip of clean cotton fabric
Nettle	Rich in iron, this blood purifier stimulates the production of fresh blood cells. It is good for all skin complaints resulting from toxins, sluggish circulation or elimination. Take as a tea during menstruation to guard against anaemia
Parsley	This cleansing herb is high in iron. Add to meals and juices
Peppermint	This stimulating digestive is often taken as an after-dinner drink. Very warming in the winter, it is useful if bowel movements are sluggish

Red sage	The herb of choice to treat all sore throats. Take as a gargle to ease throat complaints, and as a mouth-wash for ulcers and sore gums. Drink the tea (no more than one cup per day) to ease upper bronchial complaints
Rosemary	Antiseptic and cleansing, this is used in cooking and as an inhalant for breathing difficulties (particularly sinus conditions). As a tea it is a good headache cure, and will help relieve muscle cramping and spasm. Useful as an anti-fungal treatment
Slippery Elm	This is a powerfully soothing demulcent. Make it into a paste with a little water or apple juice and drink immediately to sooth the whole digestion. Useful for tummy upsets and irrated bowel
St John's Wort	This cheery herb is excellent for the skin. Soak the leaves in oil for a preparation to paint on varicose veins to bring instant relief, and for speedy healing of bruises and rough skin
Yarrow	Promotes sweating, aids kidney function, and promotes production of fresh blood cells in the bone marrow. Add to a Sitz bath to aid elimination through the kidneys. Take as a tea for cystitis, and to relieve diarrhoea

Calendula or marigold is an excellent skin healer and its cleansing action makes it suitable for use anywhere on the body. I often recommend adding it to the bath as a remedy for any vaginal infection:

Take 4oz of dried calendula and add to 1 gallon of water. Allow to steep for 12 hours and then bring to a gentle boil. Simmer for six minutes then strain the liquid into a hot bath and discard the flower heads. Sit in the bath, ensuring the kidney area is immersed, for about twenty minutes, then wrap up and go straight to bed.

A macerated cabbage leaf is another tremendous skin-cleanser – its leeching effect makes it a useful poultice for boils or deep spots:

Place a cabbage leaf in boiling water for 30 seconds (larger, more sinewy leaves may need up to 45 seconds). Place the leaf directly onto the spot, as hot as is tolerable, or if the skin is broken apply between two pieces of thin gauze. Cover with a warm bandage or towel and leave in place for up to two hours. This can be repeated as necessary.

A very old-fashioned remedy is to crush some fresh comfrey leaves and place as a compress or add to the splint for a broken bone. The comfrey or bone-knit would also be taken internally with a meal, or as a tea, to facilitate healing.

Finding out more
Dr Christopher School of Natural Healing
19 Park Terrace
Stoke on Trent
Staffordshire
British Herbal Medicine Association
Lane House
Cowling
Keighley
West Yorkshire, BD22 0LX

Further Reading

Kitty Campion, *Kitty Campion's Handbook of Herbal Health*, Sphere Books

Nicholas Culpepper, *Culpepper's Complete Herbal*, W. Foulsham and Co. Ltd

Richard Mabey (cons. ed.), *The Complete New Herbal*, Gaia/Elm Tree

Maria Treben, *Health from God's Garden*, Thorsons.

HOME REMEDIES

One of the joys of natural healthcare is that so many of the remedies and techniques for supporting full health are available to us all. Everyday articles and substances from your kitchen cupboard can provide a safe and effective cure for common ailments, and the addition of some herbs and flowers can make a full natural first-aid chest. It makes perfect sense to look here, and to the garden for simple remedies to treat everyday complaints.

During the summer months, **vinegar** and **bicarbonate of soda** are useful for treating the site of wasp and bee stings – vinegar for wasps, and bicarb for bees. Apply diluted in water to relieve the pain. Vinegar also makes a useful, cooling wash for any areas of sunburn: add one cup of vinegar to a bowlful of tepid water, and use to wash the affected area. Applying cold fresh **yoghurt** will help cool and sooth the area if the site of burning is small, and you can also use freshly sliced **tomatoes** straight from the fridge – this is especially useful on the face.

Minor burns like those you get from touching the oven shelf with a finger, will respond well to being held in a bowlful of warm water, until all the pain subsides (care must be taken, though, not to treat large burns in this way). If you get a burn on your tongue from eating or drinking something that was too hot, take a mouthful of full-fat milk and hold it in your mouth for a few minutes, swishing it around. This will work more effectively than anything else I know.

Sea salt makes a useful cleansing agent for women when added to the bath water, and has many other bath-room uses (see Skincare, pp. 285–8). Vinegar, too, can be added to help restore vaginal acidity. Add one capful of apple cider vinegar to the bath once a week for best effects.

Fresh lemons have myriad uses and in every respect naturally or organically grown ones are better than those grown chemically. Squeeze a few drops of lemon juice directly onto a cold sore or mouth ulcer for an instant, if stinging, cure. Repeat five times a day, and it will disappear within 48 hours. Squeeze lemon juice on to a wart and leave to dry in the sun, repeating as many times as you can, and it will disappear within a week. Add a few drops of lemon juice to a cup of warm water for a refreshing, alkalinizing early-morning drink that will help remedy any over-indulgences the previous night.

Water is a tremendously effective healing tool, and can be used in any number of ways. (See Hydrotherapy, pp. 139–49) A straightforward steam inhalation is a remarkably fast-acting remedy for sinus complaints, coughs, colds, and upper bronchial complaints. It is also a useful beauty treatment for the face, and can be used to treat skin complaints like acne.

Add boiling water to a large bowl and bend your head over it, covering your head and the bowl with a large towel to stop the steam from escaping. Breathe in through your nose as well as through your mouth, and try to stay under the towel for as long as possible. If you get too hot, lift your head out from time to time for a breath of cooler air, but leave the bowl covered so that none of the steam is lost.

Add a variety of botanicals to the water to enhance the effectiveness of the steam, and to add further antiseptic and cleansing qualities. **Rosemary** is particularly antiseptic, and a stem of the fresh herb rubbed between the fingers (to release its aromatic oil) and then added to the water will bring speedy relief to chesty coughs and will also loosen sinuses. One drop of the essential oil of rosemary could be used instead, or one drop of olbas oil. Rosemary is also a great astringent, so those with oily skin or pimples will benefit from this inhalation, which can be repeated daily.

Red sage is another herb which lends itself to being used in this way. It will cleanse and tone the mucous membranes and is particularly useful for soothing sore throats. This is a relative of common sage, most often used for its culinary benefits.

White thyme and **ti tree oil** are more forceful in their action, and one drop of either of these essential oils added to the inhalation will make an excellent first-aid step for any virus conditions. **Peppermint** and **eucalyptus essential oils** are effective at clearing stuffy noses and at shifting a dry cough. A few rose petals or a drop of essential oil of **rose** make a soothing inhalation which is particularly good for softening a wind- or sun-dried skin, and you could also add a few drops of **aloe vera juice**.

Poultices, packs and **compresses** are useful ways to apply the effects of water to a specific body part, and they can also be added to, or substituted by, everyday substances, herbs, essential oils and flower remedies. A simple brown bread poultice is wonderful for drawing any toxins from the skin, and can be made easily and quickly by pouring boiling water on to a bowl of crustless bread, and wringing it out. Place on a strip of cotton fabric, and apply to the area as hot as can be tolerated. Leave in place for up to four hours, replacing up to three times a day.

Poultices can be hot or cold, and the simplest one of all is to apply a fresh vegetable like potato, cabbage or onion to the skin in order to cleanse or draw out any local impurities. Apply an onion that has been cut in half onto the back of the neck, to relieve the pain of toxic headache. Cover the area first with a thin smear of sesame or olive oil, to make sure it does not irritate the skin. Wrap around with a clean tea-towel or strip of cotton fabric, and leave in place for up to two hours.

To make a hot poultice, warm some water in a non-aluminium saucepan, and add, for instance, a large cabbage leaf or some fresh sage leaves. Spread the resultant mush onto a strip of cotton gauze and wrap around the affected area with a clean tea-towel or strip of cotton fabric. This is very useful for relieving joint and arthritic pain, and can be kept warm by covering with a hot water bottle. Repeat every two hours, and then leave in place overnight to absorb the benefit of the herb.

A compress is usually applied for a very short time, and is a useful way to treat burns, stings, bruises and minor cuts. Again it can be used hot or cold, and is made by simply holding a strip of cotton fabric under the hot or cold tap, wringing out, and applying to the affected area. Add two drops of Rescue Remedy before applying to soothe and calm the area. This is especially good for bruises, and where there has been any shock. Add two drops of essential oil of lavender to the compress just before applying to relieve the pain of insect bites and stings.

Herbal tea bags make an excellent instant compress, and used ones can be kept in the fridge for an hour before applying for a refreshingly cool and astringent effect. Use chilled chamomile or peppermint on your eyes to refresh and soothe them, and nettle to soothe irritated skin. Warm rosehip placed directly on a bruise will aid resolution.

Fruit and **vegetable slices** can also be used in this way, and two cucumber rings placed on the eyes will reduce any puffiness, and freshly grated apple will sooth a rash from nettles or other plants.

Cold packs are a wonderful way to soothe a painful sprain or strain, and will help reduce any swelling, slow the inflammation process, and reduce pain. This is an excellent first-aid measure for back pain of any kind, and is what I suggest to most of my patients. The simplest method is to use a packet of frozen peas, corn, or other small vegetables. Take them from the freezer, mark them in some way with a felt-tip so that they will not be eaten, and place them straight onto the affected area. If it is too painful to the skin, then wrap in a clean tea-towel first. Leave in place for 20 minutes, and then return them to the freezer to get cold again. Repeat the application every two hours until you can get help, or every hour if the pain continues to be severe.

Further Reading

Mark Mayell, *Off-the Shelf Natural Health: How to Use Herbs and Nutrients to Stay Well*, Boxtree

Ros Trattler, ND, DO, *Better Health through Natural Healing*, Thorsons

Belinda Grant Viagas, *Natural Remedies for Common Complaints*, Piatkus.

HYDROTHERAPY

*Colonic irrigation • Drinking water • Flotation tanks •
Inhalations • Jacuzzis • Showers • Douches • Enemas •
Rebirthing • Sitz baths*

Water is a tremendously powerful therapeutic agent. It can be used internally, and externally, applied hot, warm or cold for its thermal qualities; under pressure, for partial immersion or local use. This natural therapy has been used for centuries, and its immediate effectiveness and ease of application make it a valuable tool for home healthcare. See also Home Remedies (pp. 134–5).

It is important to provide our bodies with sufficient water each day, and drinking fresh, clean water is the fastest, most effective way to do this. Unfortunately, this is not available to us in many countries, including Britain, so it needs to be filtered, or passed over in favour of bottled mineral waters.

Water has a myriad of external uses too – making use of its thermal qualities, cold packs and compresses have an immediate first-aid application for injuries. Applying a cotton cloth (tea-towel or handkerchief) that has been soaked in cold water to a muscle spasm or bruise has instant beneficial effects. The cold encourages the body to rush fresh blood supplies to the area; this brings additional oxygen and nutrients to the site so that the body can then begin its process of repair. (See Home Remedies, p. 137)

Steam inhalations, an old-fashioned remedy, are often used to relieve chest congestion, and these are particularly beneficial for any skin complaints as well as providing help and relief for sore throats and mucous conditions. You can buy facial saunas at any electrical shop, but these are not necessary in order for you to benefit fully from this treatment. You can do it yourself quite easily with a kettle, a bowl and a towel.

Regular, plain steam inhalations can form an important part of the treatment of any bronchial complaint, and can be useful in the treatment of asthma. If it is not possible to perform the procedure as advised, then the steam from an open kettle, or from a running hot-water tap can still be of assistance. In a small room, with the doors and windows closed, this steam will be inhaled, and can help make breathing easier. A person with any breathing difficulty may well be feeling anxious, however, and shutting them in like this should not be attempted if there are any feelings of claustrophobia or insecurity.

The use of **showers** or shower sprays is a valuable addition to the treatment of any part of the body. By varying the temperature of the water, your body will be encouraged to speed up the general circulation, and fresh nutrients will quickly be brought to the area being sprayed. This is particularly effective in speeding up the resolution of bruises, and hastens the recovery time of any sprains or strains. It can also relieve pelvic congestion when used on the abdominal area, or act as a general circulation enhancer if used all over on a regular basis.

The golden rule when varying the temperature of the water is always to finish with cold; so when spraying, start with warm water, then switch to cold for one minute, then back to warm, then cold again for another minute. This can be repeated up to five times, making sure to end with a cold spray, and the whole process can be repeated up to three times each day.

If a shower head is not available, the same effect can be achieved with two bowls of water, one hot and one cold, or even (if the body part is small) by holding it directly under the taps.

Another wonderfully invigorating use of shower sprays is as something strangely called a **Scottish douche**. A high pressure shower head is aimed along the length of the spine, using first hot water, then cold. This directly stimulates the nerves as they leave the bony protection of the spine and move to supply the rest of the body. The easiest way to achieve this is with someone else's help, although with careful positioning of the shower head and by moving yourself up and down, it can be done on your own. The dramatic effects are felt straightaway, and it is advisable to allow a few minutes' rest immediately afterwards, and not to do this more than once a day, unless resting.

Vaginal douches have encountered some bad press in recent years, but this is mainly as a result of their incorrect use. The only safe douche is a gravity one – this uses the pull of gravity to govern the flow of liquid and its exit from the body. The absence of any pressure or force ensures that no damage is done to the delicate vaginal walls and that the cervix will remain untroubled. The douche comprises a bag or rigid container which is filled with water or water mixed with other substances, and hung on a shower rail or wall hook; a longish tube that runs from it, and a small, removable nozzle with small perforations at its end. While standing or crouching in the bath, the nozzle is inserted into the vagina and a slow, steady flow flushes the water through and out of the body. Douches are obtainable from any chemist.

A douche solution made of nine parts warm water to one part apple cider vinegar can be dramatically helpful in the treatment of vaginal thrush, and the use of tepid water can help improve the tone of vaginal muscles after pregnancy or great weight loss. (Care must be taken at all times, and particularly after pregnancy, when this should not be performed without first checking with a healthcare practitioner.)

Douching is hopelessly ineffective as a means of contraception, often having the reverse effect and making conception more likely. It can, though, be a useful adjunct to overall healthcare, and some women find it especially useful in restoring their body's delicate balance after the use of contraceptive creams and gels.

Enemas work in essentially the same way, and most douche kits will include a separate nozzle for insertion into the anus. When using enemas, the same amount of care is needed as for douching, so as not to damage the delicate lining of this sensitive area. Enemas are most often taken whilst lying down, and in the past played an important role in many medical practices. Doctors and health practitioners would recommend them, and the practice nurse would carry out the procedure in the surgery. Nowadays they are most often used at home. Their effect on clearing the bowel is dramatic, and for this reason their use is not recommended on too regular a basis. Two or three enemas should clear any particular obstructive problem, but they should not be substituted for proper dietary care. If used too frequently (more than once a month), the body can come to rely upon them, rather than using them for assistance in times of need. The enema is quite safe if gravity assisted – this means there is no pressure used, and the flow of water is governed by the rate at which it passes naturally down the pipe and into the body.

Colonic irrigation is currently gaining in popularity – this is something quite different from an enema. Here water is pumped high into the colon under pressure, and is often aerated, or has other substances added to it. I cannot stress enough the need to have one's condition properly diagnosed prior to considering this procedure, and that it must be performed by a qualified practitioner. That they have trained on the equipment used is not sufficient qualification to allow a person to treat such a delicate and important area of the body in this way. They must also have the anatomical and physiological knowledge necessary for correct diagnosis. Often this is taught as a week-end course, and it worries me tremendously.

In more general use, water as therapy has many applications. A hot bath at the end of a long day warms and relaxes the body, and provides a useful transition time before sleeping. Cold water run over the wrists on a hot day cools and calms the whole body, and an early morning paddle in cold water stimulates and wakes the body up remarkably well. There are also many 'immersion' therapies and tools available for pleasure and/or personal growth.

Vivation^{TM} or **rebirthing** is one such tool. Here, through connected breathing and the support of the practitioner, the client is assisted in releasing negative or pent-up physical and emotional patterns. The ultimate experience is to relive one's own birth, and to this end, sessions will often take place in a specially designed pool, with both practitioner and client in the water. Once the techniques have been learned, and it is possible to let go of today's reality sufficiently to allow earlier feelings to emerge, doing this in the water can simulate the warm, watery comfort of being in the womb.

Whether this is actually re-experiencing one's own birth or not, the release of hitherto unexpressed emotions is certainly a form of psychological renewal. Most often, the images which appear to the client during such a session are birth-related – tunnels with a light at the end; being expelled by some unseen force; and entering bright colourful places are common. Rebirthers or Vivation™ practitioners often require some sessions on dry land before progressing to a pool. This is to familiarize the client with the sometimes dynamic nature of the work, and to allow time for the therapeutic relationship to establish.

Once learned, the rebirthing techniques and breathing exercises can be practised alone, and many people use a morning bath to do this in, feeling that to have begun the day with such a releasing and strong emotional experience prepares them for most eventualities.

It is very important that there is strong counselling or psychotherapeutic support while undertaking this kind of work, because of its dynamic and effective nature. To release feelings that are deep-seated, or that have been around for a long time can be a remarkable experience, but it can also be frightening. It is very important to be able to put such feelings or memories into a safe, productive perspective, and to feel not just relief, but also security after such an episode. For the maximum benefit to be gained from such releases, they need to be both understood and integrated into present reality, so always check your rebirther's training and experience before embarking on any experiential work.

Many people are now discovering the joys and benefits of **flotation tanks**. These are rather like large, enclosed baths, which are filled with warm water and epsom salts, and allow the body to simply float. Each tank is a light-proof, sound-insulated shell which contains about ten inches of water. The combination of silence, darkness and floating in the warm water generate a deep relaxation, often within minutes of entering the tank. Many people believe that re-experiencing this womb-like situation provides enormous psychological benefits.

Current research shows that the level of relaxation engendered in this environment has deep and lasting effects on stress levels, and can positively influence pain tolerance; this is mainly due to the high levels of natural pain-killers which the body is stimulated to produce. The warm, soothing nature of the experience is extremely comforting, and in allowing the conscious mind to relax, encourages the development of our more intuitive, creative side. Although most often used for relaxation, flotation tanks provide an ideal situation for creative problem solving, visualization work and other forms of self-healing. Extraordinary rates of accelerated learning have been noted, using in-tank audio or visual tapes.

The use of flotation tanks can be as regular or intermittent as needed; sometimes more than once a week feels necessary – if working with high levels of stress, for example – while at other times a monthly visit can be just enough to keep in touch with the inner calm that is experienced during a float.

Most sessions last an hour, at the end of which the floater is made aware of the time. This is often achieved by music being piped into the tank, before the door is opened. Floaters are not locked in – it is possible to leave at any time, although the most common response is one of surprise that the float is over; people will often say that it feels as though they lost track of time altogether, and that it could have been only a few minutes since they entered the space.

The presence of the salts in the water reduces any risk of infection as well as enabling you to float. Before entering, people are requested to shower, and to cover any broken skin with plasters or vaseline. The prospect of lying in bath water in which a complete stranger was lying only minutes before, however sanitized the conditions, is not a pleasing one for some people. Aside from the physical situation, there can be the feeling of entering another person's space, or being aware of their energy. To this end, flotation tank managers are usually happy to let you know when the water is changed, and to let you have a copy of their schedule of floats, so a time could be chosen at the beginning of the day, or after the tank has had a rest day. Flotation tanks can be found in a variety of health centres and beauty salons, as well as at natural health clinics and specialist float centres.

Another deeply relaxing activity is taking **jacuzzis** or **spa baths**. They ostensibly work on a more physical level – gently pummelling the body with jets and aerated water – their effects, however reach far deeper. Some people suggest that the feelings of renewal and healing that can be experienced when bathing in this way are due to subconscious memories of floating in the womb. Others posit that it is because the sea was our ancestral home, and so we are actually reaching back to some distant genetic memory.

The walk-in baths with seating areas around the side seem reminiscent of Roman bathing rituals. Stepping into the deep, warm water which can then be brought alive with the press of a button is both stimulating and relaxing. The jets can be aimed at specific body parts for an underwater pressure massage, or one can just float around, being carried in a slow circle by the whirlpool effect. Sitting with warm, swirling water bubbling up to your chin is a delightfully sensual experience.

The continuous action of the water serves as a deep massage, gently stimulating muscles and increasing overall circulation. This effect combines with the heat to have an almost intoxicating effect, and care must be taken not to stay in for too long. It is best to get out before you start to feel tired, so that the benefits can continue to be felt, rather than just leading you to want to sleep.

In countries with temperate climates, jacuzzis are often sited out of doors, and there are now whirlpool spa adjustments that can be made to regular baths in individual homes, but in the main they are situated at health clubs, gyms and leisure complexes.

Home Applications

The **sitz bath** is a wonderful way of invigorating the whole body; improving the circulation and the immune system, and relieving the nervous system. It is particularly useful in conditions of pelvic congestion or if there are any lower back problems. It is a very stimulating process, and it may be tiring, so always be sure to take a short rest afterwards.

You will need a large bowl, that is big enough to sit in – a baby bath is ideal. This is filled with cold water, and placed in a bath filled with about 12 inches of hot water. The idea is to sit in one temperature, making sure that the water covers the hips up to the waist completely, with ones feet immersed in another temperature. After one or two minutes, change places, so that the pelvis is now in hot water, and the feet in cold. Make at least one more change over, and finish with the pelvis in cold water, the feet in hot. Whilst bathing, make sure the whole pelvic area is covered by splashing water up over the abdomen and between the legs. Finish off with a brisk towel rub, and allow a short time to relax after this dynamic treatment.

Finding out more
British Rebirth Society
18a Great Percy Street
London WC1
Tel: 0171 833 0741

Holistic Rebirthing Institute
23 Albany Terrace
Leamington Spa
Warwickshire
Tel: 01926 882494

Incorporated Society of British Naturopaths
Kingston
The Couch House
293 Gilmerton Road
Edinburgh EH16 5UQ
Tel: 0131 664 3435

Further Reading

Henry Lindlahr, *Natural Therapeutics Volume II Practice*, C.W. Daniel Company.

IONS

The air around us is full of neutral, positive and negatively charged particles called ions. It is the negative ions which are the most beneficial; an over-abundance of positive ions contributes to a number of health concerns, mood changes and energy slumps.

The ion concentration present in the air we breathe is determined by a number of factors. Many natural elements increase the number of negative ions in the surrounding air; fire and water being two of the most effective. This explains some of the restful, invigorating nature of an evening spent in front of a real fire, and the feelings of expansion and renewal when close to a waterfall or any body of moving water. Actually, any natural environment is likely to have a more beneficial ionization than a synthetic one. Mountains have cleaner air than offices, this we could all agree, but recognizing that the ion concentration is a major factor in this state of affairs allows us to begin to redress that imbalance.

The synthetic fabric in curtains, carpets and furnishings; dust, cigarette smoke and other airborne particles; T.V. sets and vdu screens all increase the number of positively charged ions in the atmosphere. That means that all city air has high positive ion concentrations, and that just about all homes and places of work do too.

The effects of this are important in relation to health-care. Large amounts of negative ions have a lethal effect on bacteria, making for a cleaner environment. They effect the levels of various neuro-hormones in the blood and they reduce the level of histamine, giving relief to people with all manner of nervous complaints, tension and allergic responses. They also seem to affect the normal human circadian rhythm – the rise and fall of both physical and psychological energy throughout the day. Studies have shown that the energy dips previously considered as normal disappear if the environment is highly charged with negative ions.

The changes in mood and minor health complaints that people experience when there are sudden weather changes have led to detailed studies into the effect of ion concentrations on overall well-being. Negative ion readings by a waterfall average 30,000 per cubic centimetre (perhaps this contributes to the invigorating effects of a shower); in the countryside 1,500 per cubic centimetre; in the average home the level is approximately 100 per cubic centimetre.

Many people with health difficulties such as hay fever, bronchial complaints, asthma and migraines report a marked easing of their condition once the negative ion concentration in their immediate vicinity is raised. Others report the alleviation of problems like fuzzy-headedness, mild headache, catarrh and sinus difficulties when in such an environment.

A range of household ionizers can now be bought which generate negative ions into the home or workplace.

Smaller machines are also available for situation in cars and service vehicles. They usually work by neutralizing any excess of positive ions, as well as generating large numbers of negatively charged ones. These small machines run on mains electricity and can be moved easily from room to room. There are no known side effects; although a common by-product of ionizers is ozone, the amount they produce is no greater than that found in fresh air. People often let them run through the night in their bedrooms and report improvements in everything from the speed at which they can fall asleep and the quality of their dreams, to a reduction in snoring.

Most people who use ionizers report some general improvements in their health and feelings of well-being. There is plenty of evidence to attest to some of the beneficial effects that high levels of negative ions can generate, and there is every reason to suppose that redressing any imbalance in local ionization can have positive health implications.

Susbstituting natural fibres for synthetics at home, and choosing clothing made from cotton, linen, wool, etc., can make a tremendous difference too. Although we cannot all live close to a waterfall or in the middle of a wood, the more we allow nature into our homes and our lives, the better our overall health. This used to be the domain of hippies, and now each new piece of information that proves how greatly the natural world influences our health for the better, can be used in order for us all to benefit.

Finding out more
Wholistic Research Company
Bright Haven
Robin's Lane
Lolworth
Cambridge CB3 8HH
Tel: 01954 781074
Friends of the Earth
26–28 Underwood Street
London N1 7JQ
Tel: 0171 490 1555

Further Reading

Anna Kruger, *'H' is for ecoHome*, Gaia Books
David Pearson, *The Natural House Book*, Conran Octopus.

IRIDOLOGY

This is sometimes called iris diagnosis, and is a method of diagnosis through careful examination of the condition, colouring and markings of the eyes.

Iridologists look to diagnose the health of an individual by careful examination of the state of their eyes – relating particular divisions of the iris to specific body parts. The iris colour, its shape and markings all point to different aspects of life, or parts of the body. An individual's strength of will, structural integrity and the state of their liver can all be seen, using a map which divides the iris into a complex series of circles and divisions.

This method of diagnosis is often used by naturopaths and herbalists, who will take a very close look at the condition of the iris either through shining a light into the eye and using a small magnifying glass, or by photographing it. A photograph provides a lasting record, and also enables the subject to see the practitioner's findings. It also means that it can be compared with another photograph, perhaps six months or a year after treatment, and it will clearly show any changes. Otherwise, they will be noted on a chart of the eye, which can then be discussed.

People are often surprised at the amount of detail there

exists in their own eyes, and the iridologist will draw attention to the shape of the pupil (it can be flattened in parts by the presence of spinal misalignment), the mixture of colours, and the presence of specks or patches of white, or other colours.

Nobody really knows for certain how these patterns and colourings are formed, but there seems little doubt that they can be accurate mirrors of health, and this is perhaps best evidenced by noting the changes that can occur in the eye through life-style changes and courses of treatment. I first visited an iridologist a day before starting a detoxification programme. When I saw her again, six weeks later, she was able to show me the changes in the clarity of my eyes, and the difference in some of the markings. Although many physical changes take some time to show in the iris, some can be seen within a matter of weeks. Perhaps most useful for preventative care is the fact that general stress and the very early signs of organ distress can be seen, alongside any constitutional or genetic weaknesses or imbalance.

Although this form of diagnosis does not take the place of a case history, it provides a thoroughness and depth that make it a valuable assessment tool. It can point the practitioner towards areas of imbalance that are not yet showing symptoms, and also fill in any gaps in the patient's memory – people often forget to mention operations or illnesses which may be important in reaching a full diagnosis.

Iridology was first 'discovered' by a physician, Dr Ignatiev von Peckzely, in the nineteenth century. He noticed that an owl he was nursing with a broken wing had a dark spot in its eye, and this led him to investigate the correlation between the changes in this spot as the wing healed, and the markings in human eyes. In fact, Hippocrates mentions markings in the eyes, and physicians through the ages have noted being able to see the condition of various organs in this way.

Various maps have been developed to chart these markings, often showing slight variation, but today most people agree on the positioning of each part of the body and the relevance of particular signs and changes. There are, however, different schools of thought as to the colour representations in the eye – some take white markings to be signs of healing, others as an indication of over-stimulation, or an accumulation of unnatural substances. There is also some discussion as to the presence of inter-pretable psychological and emotional factors in the iris, and on how best to use this information. An experienced practitioner will tend to base their belief on their experiences, whatever their particular training.

Iris maps are readily available – one is reproduced here – but care must be taken if you decide to take a closer look at your own eyes. They are very light sensitive and can be easily damaged if the light you use is too strong.

Iridology is a diagnostic tool rather than a form of treatment, so how many visits you will need to make to the practitioner and how long a course of treatment takes will vary according to the type of practitioner you choose. In general, it is used by naturopaths, a number of herbalists and nutritional advisors, although its use is becoming more widespread as its effectiveness and accuracy are proven. As a general rule, once progress is being made with a particular course of treatment, an annual check-up with iridology

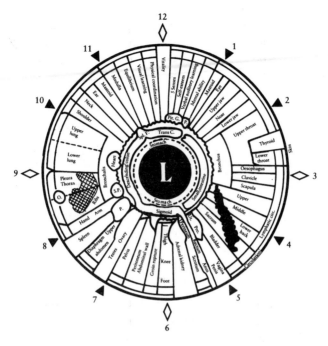

The Iris Map – Left Eye
(mirror image of one's own left eye)

is recommended to review overall health and to assess
progress.

Finding out more
National Council and Register of Iridologists
40 Stokewood Road
Swinton
Bournemouth BH3 7NC
Tel: 01202 529793

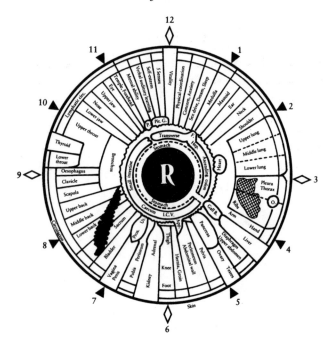

The Iris Map – Right Eye
(mirror image of one's own right eye)

British School of Iridology
Dolphin House
6 Gold Street
Saffron Walden
Essex CB10 1EJ

Further Reading

Dorothy Hall, *Iridology: How the Eyes Reveal Your Health and Personality*, Angus and Robertson

Adam J. Jackson, *Iridology: A Guide to Iris Analysis and Preventive Health Care*, Optima

Bernard Jensen DC ND, *The Science and Practice of Iridology*, BiWorld Publishers, Provo, Utah

Henry Lindlahr, *Natural Therapeutics Vol IV Iridiagnosis*, C.W. Daniel Company.

JUICING

Fresh fruit and vegetable juices are delicious, quick and easy to prepare, and packed full of goodness. Juicing extracts the beneficial minerals, vitamins and essential ingredients from plants and serves them in a tasty, easy, and quickly digestible form. Juices have many specific therapeutic uses and can form a valuable addition to an everyday diet.

In some Middle Eastern countries, particularly those where alcohol is forbidden by the religious culture, juicing has been elevated to an art form! There, exotic combinations of fresh mangoes, papaya, kiwi, guava, and other tropical and sub-tropical fruit are blended together in a delicious alternative to alcohol and carbonated soft drinks (and one that you can reproduce in your own kitchen). In a warmer climate, the need to regulate the body's fluid balance is essential, and fruit and vegetable juices can play an important part in ensuring adequate intake of water. The sense of this lesson can be applied whatever the weather.

A number of good domestic juice extractors are now on the market. Some exciting combinations can be made in a liquidizer, but a proper juicer can soon become an essential and much loved piece of kitchen equipment. Just about anything can be juiced from dandelion leaves (helpful for fluid retention) to the humble but wonderful-tasting carrot (a good source of vitamin A).

The difference between fresh juices and those available commercially is astounding; you can really taste the difference in freshness and flavour and, of course, all the vitamins and minerals are still present in the juice, along with some valuable fibre.

Vegetable juices can be substituted for a meal at any time, and make a tasty and nutritious supplement to any snack. Any variety of raw fresh vegetables can be used, except garlic – the essential oil released is so pungent, its flavour tends to linger in the machine for a long time. Carrot and celery make an excellent base – or a refreshing juice on their own. Add lettuce, a little parsley, fennel or whatever else you fancy to make a delicious range of healthy drinks.

Juicing means that the nutrients present in foods can be quickly utilized within the body. They require little energy to process, and enable rapid absorption of the vitamins and minerals they contain. Juices are ideal for providing specific nutrients, and allow the digestive system to rest. An occasional day spent on vegetable juices alone gives the body a rejuvenating fillip – supplying lots of essential nutrients and giving the body a day off from its usual digestive tasks. This frees up all the energy that is normally spent on dealing with the foods we eat, and means it can be used for other valuable jobs in the body.

Juicing also provides an alternative way of obtaining the beneficial properties from plants and herbs.

Many naturopaths recommend juices for short

cleansing diets, or when the body is in need of a rest. They also serve as an excellent introduction to whole foods after any form of fasting. When taking only juices, the stomach receives just one kind of food, and one which requires little digesting or processing before it is able to be assimilated. This makes for instant energy, and is of tremendous benefit to those with health difficulties like poor absorption.

Juices are the ideal way to provide nourishment during periods of convalescence, and at times when the appetite is low. If used specifically for health purposes, then organically grown produce should really be used. Many years ago I spent a month eating only food that had been naturally or organically grown. I then prepared a juice made from chemically grown fruits. I could taste a number of unpleasant flavours, and felt quite sick afterwards. The pesticides and other chemicals present in foods grown this way enter the body much more quickly when taken as part of a juice, and those sensitive to such additives should always choose organics.

Mixed fruits make a wonderful juice breakfast, or a sweet drink at any time of day. Try pineapple and apple as a base, and add any other fruit with the exception of bananas. Bananas will not yield juice in most extractors, and are best liquidized with a little apple juice or other fruits. During summer the wide range of berries and soft fruits makes for some wonderful combinations, but a simple winter juice of apple, pears and lemon or grapefruit is an all-round winner.

A handful of young nettles or parsley mixed with other vegetables for juicing can provide the body with much needed iron, and both are good skin cleansers. Fifteen drops of juiced mistletoe leaves taken each day is an age-old remedy to increase fertility. (Care must be taken if picking mistletoe leaves because the berries are poisonous.) Adding some fresh red peppers to a juice means extra vitamin A, and raw beetroot will give the liver a tonic.

A day on freshly juiced apples mixed with live goat's yoghurt is an excellent tonic for people with digestive difficulties, and a combination of pineapple and apple makes a refreshing cleanser, especially for meat eaters. Whisk a small glass full of the yoghurt into the juice as soon as it is extracted for a wonderfully healthy variation on a milk shake. Mixed cucumber, carrot and lettuce juice can be very helpful for people suffering with mild fluid retention, and the addition of some beetroot, celery or dandelion leaves will help accelerate the process.

When starting to include juices in your diet, begin by taking them in place of a snack, or as a pre-breakfast drink. If you are going to substitute a juice for a meal, make sure that you choose carefully in order to provide a good range of nutrients, or to provide a desired effect. Chew your juice a little, rather than swallowing it straight away, especially if it is mainly or wholly vegetable. Endeavour to juice only the best quality fruit and vegetables, and those that are as freshly picked as possible. Three days spent in storage or travelling is a long time in the life of some vitamins and the therapeutic properties of all plants are at their height when the plant is alive and growing.

If choosing to follow a juice fast for health reasons, or to aid digestion or speed some form of elimination or detox, then follow the guidelines below:
- Never follow a juice fast for more than three days without the advice and monitoring of your healthcare practitioner
- Make sure to drink large amounts of good, clean water as well as your juices. If you feel cold, drink warm water
- Take a glass of juice at least every four hours
- Take care to chew the juice a little before swallowing each mouthful, and drink it slowly
- Choose what type of juice you will have, and stick to it throughout each day – if you crave variety, choose a mixed juice
- If at all possible prepare for your juice fast carefully by eating a simple cleansing diet the day before
- Break your juice fast carefully by reintroducing solid foods slowly. The longer the juice fast, the greater care your digestive system deserves. Begin with one of the foods that you have been taking as a juice, and if that sits well with you, eat another piece one hour later. After that, begin to mix your fruits or vegetables, or introduce different types, and then progress to cooked foods.

> Taking a juice day once a month, or even once every week during the warmer weather, is a wonderful way to reinforce your health, and provides a good source of instantly available energy. It is one of the most enjoyable health-care measures.

Finding out more
Incorporated Society of British Naturopaths
Kingston
The Coach House
293 Gilmerton Road
Edinburgh EH16 5UQ
Tel: 0131 664 3435
The Soil Association Ltd
86–88 Colston Street
Bristol, BS1 5BB
Tel: 01272 290661

Further Reading

The Complete Raw Juice Therapy, Thorsons
Bernard Jensen, *Doctor–Patient Handbook*, Bernard Jensen Enterprises, California.

KINESIOLOGY

Applied Kinesiology • Touch for Health

Kinesiology, or **Applied Kinesiology** (AK), was devised by an American chiropractor, Dr George Goodheart, in 1965. It is essentially a system of muscle testing, the results of which can be said to point to any deficiencies in organ function and general health. It was devised as an adjunct to chiropractic work, to correct structural imbalances and as an aid to diagnosis.

The large muscle groups are initially tested for their strength and uniformity of response, and smaller individual muscles may then be tested to pin-point any dysfunction. These are then treated by the use of massage and pressure on specified points which relate to the meridians, or energy pathways, within the body. Any weaknesses can also point towards nervous impairment resulting from spinal misalignments. This is really a very simple way of asking the body what is wrong with it, and allowing the body to respond physically – by withdrawing its energy or amplifying it to answer as yes or no.

The system is really a synthesis of the best of Eastern tradition (the energy map) and manipulative therapy, with an anatomical base. The muscles which lie on the path that the meridian is said to take through the body are related to the organ which governs that meridian. So, a poor muscle response on the liver meridian as it passes through the shoulder area may point to a lower than normal liver energy, which can be improved through strengthening that muscle.

AK is nowadays also used for allergy testing, on the basis that if an allergy is present, the body will not be working effectively. This form of testing is used by a number of bodyworkers and some nutritionists, and a growing number of dentists now use it to assess sensitivity to mercury amalgam fillings.

The classic test is to have the patient stand with one arm extended. The practitioner will pull down on this arm, against the patient's resistance, and assess its strength. An amount of a test substance, often chalk or another mineral, will then be held in the patient's other hand while the test is repeated, and there should be no change in the response. The substance will then be replaced by a piece of amalgam (or other suspected allergen) while the test is repeated once more. In the case of a sensitivity, the arm will appear much weaker, falling easily under the same pressure which it had just resisted.

The tests can also be used to confirm the benefits of some substances, and have been used to demonstrate the positive effects of crystals on the individual's energy. Holding a crystal for a short period of time can be seen to strengthen the test response, without the body being worked on at all. This again demonstrates the battery-type effect of quartz and other crystals, which can recharge or balance a person.

People are often surprised at the intensity of their response to these seemingly simple techniques; and this is an important factor in confirming their effectiveness. It would be too simple to suggest that the changing response is totally due to psychological factors, or mind over matter, or that changes in effectiveness could occur as the muscle becomes tired. The testing does seem to accurately reflect the body's condition, and the experience is so strong that most people are convinced of that after just one try.

AK muscle testing can also be used to check for vitamin and mineral deficiencies. The patient touches a body part relating to the nutrient with one hand, while the other arm is tested. The need for B vitamins, for example, can be measured with the patient touching the tip of their tongue. (This is because the B vitamin complex needs to be spelled out, one specific vitamin at a time.)

Since its inception, AK has branched further into behavioural kinesiology (created by John Diamond to concentrate on environmental and life-style factors) and **Touch for Health**. Behavioural kinesiology has added an emotional aspect to the treatment, and has proved a valuable form of testing for environmental allergies. Touch for Health was devised by John F. Thie for use by the lay person. He intended its use to provide the opportunity for families to share a new kind of touching – one that is healing rather than invasive or sexual.

Touch for Health is a simplified form of AK and one that can easily be used by individuals in their own homes. It forms the basis for the muscle testing described previously, and includes straightforward forms of treatment and assessment. Touch for Health also includes a more energetic focus, and contains many techniques to specifically address energy imbalances.

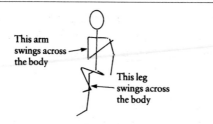

This arm swings across the body →

This leg swings across the body ←

Cross crawling is a wonderfully invigorating kinesiology exercise. It has been seen to improve co-ordination between the right and left hemispheres of the brain, and as such has proved important in the treatment of children with impaired development. Its use for adults is as a refreshing, enlivening exercise, and one that can improve concentration and relieve weariness. You can do this every morning to tone the body and mind, and to unite them in their purpose, or use this as a quick pick-me-up at the end of the day, or whenever you need an energy boost. Regular use shows some positive results in terms of improved co-ordination and greater awareness.

Stand upright with feet shoulder-width apart, and begin to 'march' on the spot. Lift your knees quite high and bring them slightly in towards the midline with each lift, extending them back to their original place as you put your feet down.

Swing your left arm across your body as your right knee comes up, and back as your right foot is replaced. Swing your right arm across your body as your left knee comes up, and back as your left foot is replaced. This is a complicated thing to describe in words, but is very simple to do. Imagine yourself wanting to cross a midline point in your body with both your upper and lower limbs. To keep a good rhythm, you use your right arm with your left leg.

Testing for allergies

To do this most effectively you will need a friend or family member to help you. Gather a small selection of everyday food-stuffs, and things you come into contact with regularly, including any that you suspect you may have an allergy towards. If you can make them all the same size it will be easier to test for them – if not you could place them all in a small brown paper bag, or a glass dish, to hold. If you are using either of these, you will need to test that you do not have a problem with that substance on its own, before you use it to contain any other objects.

The basic testing will be the same for each substance, and it is probably best to limit your testing to a maximum of one dozen different substances at any one time. Stand up straight, and raise your right arm up into the air in front of you, and slightly out to one side. Make a loose fist, and keep your hand at a level a few inches above your head. Take the object (or hold the bag or dish) in your left hand, close your hand around it, and hold it to your middle, close to your belly button. It is best if you do not know what the substance is, so either close your eyes, or have your tester put each item into your hand.

Take a deep breath. Now, without tensing too much, hold your right hand and arm strongly in place. Your tester is going to take a hold of your right arm about half way along your forearm, and pull down, just as they would on a pump. Not much force is used, just enough to move your arm down, and test the level of resistance that your muscles are offering. As the muscles release their pull, your arm will spring back into place. Keep it there, while you empty your left hand and another object is placed there.

Usually the level of resistance is more or less the same, until you test with a substance that is especially good for you, when the arm will feel considerably stronger, or with something that is not good for you, when the arm will go surprisingly weak. The differences are usually very noticeable, so if you sense only a slight change, consider that to be normal.

This is a very effective way of testing for allergies, but it can also be used to determine which crystals or stones may be of most benefit to your body, or which vitamins or supplements are needed. The range of applications for this is enormous, from testing for contact allergies, to wool or washing powder, for example, to whether situations or people are healthy for you at any specific time.

If you get a positive reaction for any allergens, avoid that food or substance for about three weeks, and take some extra vitamin C during that time. After three weeks expose yourself to the food or substance, and see whether you are still getting a reaction. Do not take more than three foods out of your diet at any time without the guidance of your natural healthcare practitioner or nutritional advisor. If you get a positive reaction for substances that will strengthen you, introduce them – eat them, wear them, or whatever is appropriate – for a similar period, and see if you can notice any difference in yourself. After that time, give yourself a break, and after a week's rest, re-test.

Finding out more
Association for Systematic Kinesiology
39 Browns Road
Surbiton
Surrey KT5 8ST
Tel: 0181 399 3215
Association of Systemetic Kinesiology
48 Percy Place
Ballsbridge
Dublin 4
Tel: 01 660 2806
Touch for Health Foundation
1174 North Lake Avenue
Pasadena
California 91104-3797
USA
Tel: 818 794 1181

Further Reading

John F. Thie, DC, *Touch for Health: A new approach to restoring our natural energies*, DeVorss and Company, California.

LAUGHTER

This is one of my all-time favourite natural therapies. Happiness is as important to continued good health as a heartbeat. It doesn't matter how much good food you eat, if you do not enjoy a mouthful of it, it will not be good for you. If you hate your life, what's the point in living and being well? Our attitude is all-important to the quality of daily life, and happiness and joy deserve to be cultivated and followed. If we are true to ourselves, and follow our hearts, then joy will always lead us well. From a spiritual perspective, joy is the key to our future, and a fundamentally important part of our progress.

Laughter is wonderful therapy – in every sense of the word. You can do it anywhere, and at any time; it exercises your body beautifully, promotes the release of mood-enhancing chemicals in your brain, and, depending on your timing, can infuse others with the same sense of joy and mirth.

As well as being fun to do, laughing exercises the neck, the muscles of the chest wall and the diaphragm, and ensures that the stomach and the liver, spleen and other organs are gently massaged. With the diaphragm acting as a pump, fresh nutrients and oxygen supplies are speeded around the body, and peristalsis, the way food naturally moves through the gut, is improved. Genuine laughter even increases the level of an antibody in the saliva – IGA – which helps protect against colds and flu. A regular prescription of laughter has been shown to improve recovery time after illnesses, and reduce the need for external pain relief. It is well worth seeking it out while in good health too.

Scheduling time for fun into our busy lives pays off. It is a lovely way to ameliorate some of the effects of stress, and everybody needs fun. If you stop and remember the last time you found something roaringly funny, it was probably too long ago. Take a moment right now to organize or plan a time for some fun and laughter in your life this week. It may be an evening out with friends, renting a funny video, going to see a comic or a comedy film, or buying a book of cartoons. Laughter is a very individual thing, and what tickles some people to pieces leaves others quite unmoved, so seek out your own laughter stimulus, and develop this aspect of yourself.

There is a meditation technique based on laughing, which builds on its infectious quality and as such is often most effective when used in groups, at least initially. It serves as an introduction to feeling really in touch with our true feelings and provides a good contact with the energy centre in the abdomen.

Participants start laughing, usually in response to the teacher's own laugh, and soon find it very easy to keep going, prompted by the laughter around them. At a given point, they stop, and immediately close their eyes and focus their attention in the centre of their bodies. The release of emotion through laughter makes for easy access to the stillness which is to be found within all of us. The participants' responses are all about recognizing that calm, and contacting feelings of joy, stillness and peace within themselves.

For centuries we have known about the importance of our state of mind and its connection with good health. An optimistic attitude truly is a life saver, and finding humour in a situation can provide a myriad of immediate benefits too.

A simple smile can positively affect your health. The facial muscles exert a direct influence on an area in the brain called the limbic system. This group of glands acts as a switchboard, regulating the speed that nerve impulses are transmitted and thereby controlling the level of performance of both mind and body. All the nerve messages from throughout the body must pass through this system and the effect of smiling is to speed their passage by increasing the number of neurotransmitters, the chemicals which carry the messages.

An inner smile is a wonderful thing to cultivate. You can do this for the good feelings it engenders, or as part of a meditation practice. Do this every day for a week, and notice the effect it will have on your life.

1. Sit quietly, feeling calm and relaxed. Make sure that your spine is straight, and that you are not experiencing any restriction from tight clothes. Take a deep, comfortable breath, and as you breathe out, imagine any tension and disharmony

---

leaving your body. Repeat this a few times, then return to your normal, relaxed, rhythmic breathing. Close your eyes, and go within yourself.

2. Without moving or opening your eyes, start to smile with your eyes. Let them fill with the softness and gladness that you would normally feel if you were really smiling, and be aware of the skin around your eyes relaxing and softening too. Let them stay smiling while you go on and smile with your pituitary gland. This is about the size of a walnut, and is situated right in the middle of your head, behind your nose. Feel this soften and expand as you allow it to smile, and see that as it does so, a single drop of precious golden elixir begins to fall from it.

3. This carries a message to the rest of your hormonal system to keep working in time and rhythm. Watch as the drop, thick and viscous, hangs there in all its richness, and then slowly in all its glistening glory slides down. You can catch it on the very back of your tongue, and you will almost be able to taste it. Enjoy the feeling as this golden syrup reaches your tongue, and touches it with a magic of its own. Feel your tongue express your own inner smile as it softens and gently curls up at the edges to fill your mouth more comfortably.

4. The golden drop then glides down your throat, and everywhere it passes smiles with the joy of knowing it is there. Feel as your throat and neck expand slightly, and relax into their most comfortable position.

5. Your eyes are still smiling, more so now at the sight of this golden messenger and how well it is received by your body. Notice how you can smile with your shoulders, and feel

the happiness that is there. The drop falls slowly and languorously into the top of your chest, where it is received by a soft thymus gland. Feel this smile fill your chest and expand around your rib cage to your back. Notice how this sticky fluid has left a trail of sunshine behind it, and revisit the smiling and ease that exist all over your head and neck.

6. Work your way slowly and surely through all your organs, from your stomach down to your genitals, visiting each of them in turn, and letting them relax into a strong inner smile. Feel as each part of you relaxes and curls up, expanding itself and settling down to its most comfortable, joyous position. Take your time, and enjoy the feeling in every part of you as it in turn manifests your own perfect, individual inner smile, and lets go of any tension or disharmony. Feel yourself to be filled with the love that your smile expresses, and bask a while in that feeling.

7. Finish by returning to your eyes, and enjoy their secret smile for a few minutes, before slowly opening them, taking a deep breath, and stretching wherever you need to. Sit still for a few minutes to digest the feelings of this experience, and know that you can return to it whenever you choose.

MASSAGE THERAPY

Massage has been defined as 'treatment of the muscles using rubbing or kneading'. Anyone who has received a good massage can tell of the many different levels on which they felt cared for and treated. This hands–on method of working on the whole body can be used to treat muscle soreness and stiffness, but it can also do a lot more than that.

Massage techniques can be used to help individuals with specific complaints ranging from asthma and bronchitis to menstrual pain. They can be incorporated into any stress management plan for the total relaxation they help to engender, and can also be used to address a number of joint problems. They can aid suppleness in the body by break-ing down fluid retention, fatty deposits and releasing areas of immobility. Massage can also be used to access and aid in the resolution of emotional issues. Most often, though, it is seen as a treat.

On a physical level, a general massage will improve lym-phatic drainage, increase overall circulation, stimulate the nervous system and soothe the skin. It can provide an enor-mous boost of energy that will manifest itself in an easy, relaxed way. Massage can also improve communication between mind and body, and can be a tremendous aid to anybody seeking an increased physical awareness.

Most massage therapists work at health clinics and sports facilities, although some will also visit your home. The initial session will begin with the taking of a short health history – the therapist will also want to know about any specific aches and pains, and whether there are any 'trouble-spots'. We all tend to hold tensions somewhere in the body, the commonest sites are the shoulders, lower back, and stomach – these are the places that ache or get uncomfortably tight when we are stressed. If you are not aware of any particular tensions, the therapist will soon find which areas need to be worked on once the massage begins.

The therapy room might feel unusually warm to begin with, but this is important to ensure full relaxation when you are being massaged. Lying still, you tend to get cold, and the presence of oil or cream on your skin can heighten this effect. It is important for the room to be warm so that your muscles do not become too tense – this would undo many of the beneficial effects of the treatment.

Some people undress completely to receive a massage, others leave on their underwear. The therapist will be quite used to working with all sorts of bodies, so modesty need not be an issue – it is important to do whatever will feel most comfortable. Any body parts not being worked on will be covered with a towel or blanket, and this helps with the modesty question as well as providing additional warmth.

You can elect to have just a back, or a neck and shoulder massage if this is what you would prefer, although a complete treatment is most beneficial. A full body massage usually begins with a person lying on their tummy on the treatment couch, while the therapist begins work on their back. Some form of cream is most often used, although some therapists prefer to use oils. (See Aromatherapy for the use of essential oils, pp. 29–32.) One of the most wonderful aspects of this type of work is that however bright or quick-thinking you may be, it is impossible to keep track of the different techniques and pressure strokes that the therapist will use. There really is no option, then, but to surrender to relaxation, and to enjoy the pleasurable feelings. Being able to receive that amount of care in such a relaxed and secure environment is a tremendously enriching experience.

Touch has to be one of our most underused senses – usually this degree of tactile nourishment only takes place between mother and baby, or between lovers. Perhaps this is one of the reasons for the use of this word as a misnomer by escort agencies and the like. Nothing could be further from the truth for massage therapy, however, but this is one reason why many female therapists will only work on other women. Although massage therapy has nothing to do with sex or sexual massage, many women find it easier to relax, particularly while undressed, with another woman.

During a treatment, the legs and neck will also be worked on before turning the client or patient over and working over the front of the legs, the arms and hands, neck, shoulders and face. Abdomens and chests seem to be an optional extra – most therapists will ask you if you want these areas to be treated.

Although using a similar range of techniques — stroking, percussion, kneading, pummelling, etc., each massage therapist will develop their own style, so the feelings and the treatment will vary from one practitioner to another. There are also areas of speciality — some therapists concentrate on sports or remedial massage, others on relaxation, or on the beautifying aspects of improved skin tone and texture (partly from all that lovely cream or oil). Massage can also assist weight reduction by stimulating the lymphatic system and helping to break down fatty tissue. It is important to establish what type of massage you want — relaxation, for example, or to help with a training injury.

Many healers use massage, and concentrate on the more energetic aspects of the treatment. Intuitive massage therapists allow themselves to be guided to areas of tension by the feel of a client's body, rather than by following any strict anatomical pattern.

After a treatment, there is usually time to just lie still and appreciate the wonderful, warm feelings of deep physical relaxation. The therapist will be busy washing their hands and writing up your notes, and may even leave you alone for a while to gather your thoughts before you need to dress again. Many clinics and health centres have shower facilities which you can use after a treatment, but it is also nice not to have to do anything other than hold on to those positive feelings. Those lucky enough to find a visiting therapist can, of course, remain totally relaxed without having to think about any of these things.

Some massage oils can stain certain fabrics (particularly poly-cottons) so you may want to have a change of clothing with you, but your skin will have absorbed most of the cream or oil that was used.

Massage therapy courses are available at many adult education centres and at health clinics. It is very easy, though, to begin massaging yourself and friends or family without any formal training. A good shoulder rub can be a wonderful thing at the end of a busy day, and it is easy to feel any tight spots even through layers of clothing. Children love being massaged, and baby massage is a wonderfully soothing experience for both partners.

You can massage yourself anywhere except on the back. This is a lovely way to begin or end the day, and makes a wonderful after-bath treat. Simply use some cream, body lotion or oil, and begin by gently stroking whichever body part you have chosen to work on. The legs, feet, arms and abdomen all lend themselves to self-massage, and you can give yourself a wonderfully relaxing abdominal massage while lying down.

1. Gently warm any oil you are going to use, unless you are straight out of the bath, when your body heat will be sufficient. Always decant some of the cream or oil onto your hands first, and rub them together until fully lubricated, before spreading that on your skin. Keep a towel nearby in case of spills, and to wipe your hands on, and make sure that the rest of your body is kept warm and covered.

2. The massage techniques are the same for whatever part of the body you are working on. Follow the contours of your skin closely with your hands so that you feel warm and cared for. Vary the pressure and the length of each stroke that you

use, alternating light, sweeping strokes that will spread the massage cream, with shorter, deeper strokes that really pay attention to a particular feature. Simple kneading movements can be made by pressing down with your hands, and gentle pressure from your thumbs and even your knuckles can be used on fleshy areas, and on the soles of the feet.

3. Keep your strokes slow and rhythmic as you press deeper into your muscles, and let them be a little faster on more superficial strokes. Play a little, and experiment with what feels best – sometimes some areas want a little more care than others, and certain body parts may want waking up and stimulating. This is a lovely way to get to know your own body, in a way that no other medium allows you to. Allow your hands to get a full sense of the part of your body that they are working on, as well as to give pleasure and comfort.

4. Continue your massage for as long as it feels good. Never use any pressure when working on your abdomen, here the best stroke to use is a gentle circular motion, and do not ever continue if you feel any pain or discomfort. If you have a professional massage you may well pick up some tips for other techniques, but simply covering yourself with your own loving, caring touch can be remarkably therapeutic.

5. Finish your massage by gently holding whatever body part you have been working on, or resting your hands there. Let the warmth from your hands fill that area of your body, and stay there a while, breathing gently. Take your attention to that area of your body, and let yourself become aware of the gentle warmth, relaxation and good feeling that exists there. Commit that feeling to memory, so that your body will be able to replicate it for you at a later date.

You can heighten the experience by lighting some candles and turning out the lights, or playing some soothing music, or using essential oils in your massage. Perhaps you could plan an evening of sensual pleasure for yourself, and do your massage after soaking in an aromatherapy bath lit only with candles. Massage can be a useful tool in exploring this aspect of your nature.

Finding out more
Clare Maxwell Hudson School of Massage
87 Dartmouth Road
London NW2 4ER
Tel: 0181 450 6494
Irish Massage Therapists Association
Ard Lynn
Mount Rice
Monasterevin
Co Kildare
Tel: 045 525 579
The Northern Institute of Massage
100 Waterloo Road
Blackpool
Lancashire FY4 1AW
Tel: 01253 403548

Further Reading

Roberta deLong Miller, *Psychic Massage*, Harper and Row
George Downing, *The Massage Book*, Arkana.

MEDITATION

This is a wonderful method of stilling the conscious mind and allowing a 'free space'; a time of renewal and rejuvenation for the body and mind. It is a way to experience complete peace and harmony, of feeling centred deep within yourself, and of returning to the original source.

Meditation takes many forms, and different schools and philosophies advocate a variety of techniques for attaining this state. It is one of the best natural therapies. Through meditation we can approach and embrace higher levels of awareness, and enter a quiet, contemplative state that is still and untroubled by everyday thoughts and concerns. The conscious mind may then interpret the new experience, and the whole person benefits.

Some people use meditation as a form of relaxation; others to achieve 'time off' from physical and mental concerns. It can also be a powerful aid to personal growth and a deeply spiritual experience. It can be practised every day, or on an occasional basis, although a regular practice often shows best results, especially in the beginning. Many people begin their day with meditation, and sometimes meditate at the end of the day too, or in the late afternoon. Because meditation is so deeply restful, if you do it just before bed it can delay you getting off to sleep. It is a useful way to catch up with yourself if you do not have much time for sleeping.

Meditation is essentially 'still sitting' or sitting still, but the stillness is not purely physical. There is a wonderful sense of rich silence and a balmy calm to be found when the mind and awareness both become quiet. There is also a unique unity of purpose, when body and mind are joined in this way.

One technique is to systematically train the mind to be aware of different areas of the body and to recognize any local stresses. These can be consciously relaxed, and the mind is then free to float; allowing the body to recharge itself. This takes conventional relaxation skills one step further, in that the time spent after physical relaxation is achieved is perhaps the most valuable of all.

Active meditation is a unique method for problem solving. The problem, or question to be asked, is repeated over and over again either silently or out loud, and this serves to focus the individual's resources almost entirely. The repeating can be continued for a day or longer – it is important that there should be no other claims on the person's attention, so time is often a limiting factor. Suddenly, there seems to come a point when, almost like the waters of a river breaking through a surface covering of ice, the tension of holding the thought becomes almost unbearable, and an answer bubbles up from somewhere deep inside. Such moments of personal revelation can be deeply inspiring, renewing our confidence in our own inner source of wisdom.

Those following a guru or the teachings of a spiritual

leader, will often meditate with a photo of them, or while listening to the sound of their voice. This facilitates a sense of connection with their teacher and serves as a reminder of their presence or vibrations. Many gurus, in keeping with their Indian and Eastern traditions, advocate a regular practice of meditation as part of any spiritual journey or preparation for enlightenment.

The thinking behind this is based on the assumption that we all have our own unique path to follow – our own star. Only by reinforcing the connection with our own inner motivations and wisdom can we be true to ourselves, and fulfil our own promise or destiny. More immediately, this awareness of our inner selves helps us to act in ways that are right or appropriate for us. In a busy world of conflicting demands and influences, meditation can support individual integrity and clarify personal choices.

It is from a feeling of a knowledge of, and a security within ourselves, that we may reach out and embrace other experiences. Meditation can therefore be centred around uniting us with universal principles such as love or peace. Within the framework of a Teaching or Religion, the Buddha-energy or Christ-energy, for example, can be held as a model for that experience. An important point is that the focus here is on the awareness of a quality or archetype that may be touched upon to expand our own consciousness.

Mediation is not a way of escaping from reality, although it is a remarkable way of transcending our everyday experiences and reconnecting with our higher selves. The feelings can be described as being 'truly real', when we gain a clearer view of ourselves in an overall scheme of things, and rediscover what really matters to us. Some people describe reaching a place deep within themselves, others speak of sensing a place that is beyond their usual frames of reference, and different from ordinary, everyday reality.

Many psychics use a candle flame for another form of meditation which actually develops their seeing sense. Focusing on the flame, they work to alter its colour – changing it through the colours of the rainbow before reverting to seeing it as it is in this reality. The image of the candle flame can be held in the mind's eye and used in the same way. As can the symbol of a flower bud, which can be 'made' to unfold, close, open and change colours. This is a powerful way of strengthening one's psychic skills, and many psychics find themselves free to experience a meditative state quite spontaneously once their psychic energies are focused in this way.

Some people achieve meditation very easily, whenever they want or need to. For others, a regular practice is an important part of the learning process. All the techniques are really just means to an end, so one or more can be used, or they can all be experimented with before finding a way that works best for you.

Sit down in a comfortable position, making sure that your spine is straight – support it if you need to with cushions. Make sure that you will be warm enough, and that there will be no interruptions. Burning incense can encourage feelings of rest-fulness, and it is said to remind us of spirit energy in the trans-

---

formation from the material stick or cone, through the power of the flame (spirit) into something that affects us (the smell) but that we can neither see nor touch.

Plan to sit for at least twenty minutes, or half an hour at a time. You can set an alarm clock to mark the end of the meditation, but a gentle, non-jarring sound is best. Ideally, trust to your inner clock, and surrender to the knowledge that you will be able to remain in meditation only for as long as you need. Initially, the mind has a tendency to review all sorts of things. Memories and ideas seem to flood the thoughts, and it would be easy to follow any one of them. The aim of meditation is not to pay these mental workings any notice, but to centre your attention in another place – one that will not be influenced by the passing thoughts, but is able to just let them come and go. This is the position of witness or onlooker. It is non-judgemental, but is deeply rooted in a true sense of what is right. It is not rigid, but it is strong enough not to be seduced from its purpose.

When your meditation is over, rest for a moment with your eyes still closed, before coming back to everyday reality. Take a moment to review how you are feeling right now, and the way that your body feels. Take deep, refreshing breaths for a few moments, and begin to move your fingers and toes as you breathe out. Stretch, if you feel you need to, with your out breath, and then slowly open your eyes. Do not touch your face or your head for some while after meditating, and keep any movements fluid and easy, continuing the energy of the meditation and allowing it to manifest in your life.

Chants and mantras are often used to aid meditation; either as something to occupy the mind and seduce it into stillness, or for the harmonic vibration of the sound itself. You could use a positive and gentle word that has meaning for you by allowing it to repeat over and over in your mind. Love, peace, softness, care, beauty, ease, renew or refresh are all good choices.

Meditation techniques can include fixing your attention on a strong visual image, like a simple shape in a primary colour, a red circle, for example. Stare at this for some time until the image remains in front of you when you close your eyes. This will also be something on which to concentrate your mind until a deeper state is achieved. Or you could focus on an imaginary line that extends out in front of you – all the way to infinity. With your eyes closed, follow the line, and let it lead you out of your current consciousness into another state of awareness.

'OHM' is a well known mantra that can be used for meditation, but is more often spoken or sung. It means peace. This can be repeated slowly, starting with a deep in-breath, and feeling the belly of the 'O' sound coming from a place below your diaphragm. Let the sound then rise, along with your own energy, through the body and into the top of your head by the time you reach the 'M'. Hold this for a moment or two, before starting again. The effects of raising your energy up through your body in this way can be quite dynamic, and it is not unusual to feel a little light-headed after doing this for some time. This is a good way to focus yourself, and achieve some of the positive effects of meditation without actually doing it.

There are many tapes for **guided meditation** on the market that will take you to a quiet, healing place deep within yourself. You can design one of these inner journeys for yourself, and record it on to a tape to play when you are feeling quiet and relaxed.

These focusing exercises can easily transport you to wonderful surroundings where your body and mind can be nourished with beauty and touch, warmed by the sun, or moved by the rhythmic rolling of waves. The mind has amazing power over the body's responses; strongly imaging yourself to be in a place and feeling the emotions and sensations engendered can be as therapeutic as actually being there.

The simplest way to do this is to describe a situation that is peaceful, rich and renewing. It might be totally imaginary, or it might be somewhere you have been, or would like to visit. Plan your situation carefully, and remember to include all the important details, leaving room to notice new things, and experience sensations in a different way, e.g. notice any scents or aromas carried on the breeze; feel the sand between your toes; hear the rustling of the leaves. Remember to leave time between your suggestions on the tape, to allow yourself to drink in the surroundings and luxuriate in the feelings. One of the best ways to do this is to ask questions on the tape, allowing your experience to be different time after time, e.g. you can feel the sunlight on your back as you walk towards the waterfall, what is it that you hear?

Many Buddhist centres teach classes in meditation, and they can also be found at adult education centres, and natural health clinics. This simple practice is a powerful way to unite body and mind and encourage awareness of our subtle or energetic nature. It is a direct way of contacting spirit. It can also be a reminder of a time when we were not separate from the world; a reuniting with the world of spirit, or the source.

Finding out more
RIGPA Fellowship
44 St. Paul's Crescent,
London NW1 9TN
Tel: 0171 485 4342
School of Meditation
158 Holland Park Avenue
London W11 4UH
Tel: 0171 603 6116

Further Reading

Doriel Hall, *Healing with Meditation*, Gill & Macmillan.

NATUROPATHY

Nature cure, naturopathy and natural heathcare are all terms adopted to designate a system of natural healing; natural in the sense that it must be in accordance with natural law. In natural law, we look at natural or normal basic behavioural patterns, e.g. nutrition, reproduction, outdoor habit (contact with fresh air, sun, etc.), contact with water, soil and other organisms (including people); exercise, play and sleeping patterns.

There is a large range of therapies considered 'natural', including dietary therapy, massage, neuromuscular technique, osteopathy and other bodywork, hydrotherapy, clay therapy, the use of herbs, exercise, and counselling. All the therapies covered in this book, in fact. Most naturopathic trainings cover all of these topics, although the emphasis changes according to different schools of thought – some concentrating on a wide knowledge of the many available treatment forms, others concentrating on one or two modalities, and an understanding of the others.

One turn of the century catechism of nature cure defined it as: 'A system of the person building in harmony with the constructive principle in nature, on the physical, mental and moral planes of being.' Heavy with the language of that time, this does at least give an example of the comprehensive scope of natural therapy.

By the 1960s a British naturopathic association had developed the following outline: 'Naturecure is a philosophic concept on which naturopathy is founded. This concept embraces a belief in, and a full appreciation of, the self-regulating, self-adjusting and self-healing ability of the human organism, scientifically termed homoeostasis. Naturopathy is the professional practice of those therapies based upon the naturecure concept which are directed towards the releasing of the inherent healing force, therefore aiding in the restoration of the homoeostatic equilibrium and in the reversal of the disease process.'

So, the naturopath's motto is 'only nature heals', and the work is in finding ways to facilitate that healing in appropriate and non-interventionist ways. The primary objective of naturopathy is not just to cure, but to educate the patient to live in harmony with their body's unique recipe for full health. Although many of our workings are the same, individual's have different constitutional strengths, aptitudes and responses, and varied levels of vitality.

All practising naturopaths will develop their own synthesis of techniques for working with the tenets of naturopathy, although they will all cover three basic areas – the body systems, structure, and a counselling aspect. One of the most common medley of therapies is naturopathic dietary therapy and life-style advice, osteopathy or massage, and some form of counselling.

There are purists in the naturopathic world, as there are in any other aspect of life. Some would consider the use of vitamin supplements and herbal compounds as unnatural, and at the other end of the spectrum there are those who include interventionist forms of treatment such as acupuncture as part of their treatment plans. My own view is that our need for support is constantly growing in synch with the destruction of our natural resources. As the pressures upon us mount up, and industrial and other pollutants take their toll on every area of our lives, from the food we eat to the levels of noise we must endure, so our basic constitutional strengths can become eroded. Reintroducing simplicity and natural habits and cures can enable the body to right itself.

My first choice is to work with foods and lifestyle changes, things people can put into practice for themselves, and back them up with counselling and bodywork. It is important that these healthcares are well wrapped in a strong package of self-help measures to empower the individual and place them back in control of their own process. The joy of naturopathy is that it makes available so many different forms of cure; for example, if the need is great and nutrient levels are dangerously low, then vitamin and mineral supplementation is a quick way to restore some level of normal function. I do not practise any form of treatment that is invasive to the body or the psyche, and I do not personally believe that these are necessary for most people. The body's own instinctive urge is to be as well as it can, and this is a powerful ally to have in any healing plan. It is very simple and easy to encourage that in positive, beneficial ways that are health-enhancing, supportive, and truly successful.

A visit to a naturopath begins with the taking of a

comprehensive case history. The practitioner will want to know about your current life style, relationships and feelings as well as your health history. The illnesses and feelings you had as a child, and some details of your parents' health will add important building blocks to the overall picture of your own vitality and constitution; the ways in which your body copes with disease and how quickly you recover. Any operations, surgical removals (tonsils, appendix, etc.), immunizations, allergies and broken bones will also help the diagnosis.

Pharmaceuticals often block the body's own ability to cope, so particular attention will be paid to any medicines you are currently taking, or courses of drugs you have taken in the past. (Close to 98 per cent of all prescription drugs have negative side effects. Fifty per cent of prescriptions are solely to suppress symptoms, and a recent study shows 48 per cent of antibiotic courses prescribed in the last year in the UK to have been both unnecessary *and* ineffective!)

Many naturopaths will ask you to keep a diet diary for a few days prior to your first visit, to get an idea of your eating habits and to help with assessing your nutritional status. The consultation may also include some form of structural assessment, usually from an osteopathic viewpoint, and this is particularly relevant in the presence of back pain, general aches and pains or problems in a particular area of the body. Routine tests like blood pressure and pulse rate may also be carried out.

Even if you visit a naturopath with a specific health complaint, a full investigation will be made of your overall health because naturopaths maintain that illnesses do not occur in isolation; the whole person is involved. There is no point in treating a symptom without finding and treating the underlying cause. This may mean that the treatment for a stomach ulcer, for example, would involve making dietary changes, taking herbs or supplements, learning some form of relaxation technique and perhaps undertaking some counselling, or having some osteopathy; depending upon what was behind the ulcer – what caused it to occur in the first place. In this respect, naturopaths work as primary care providers, fulfilling the role of a natural GP. They can help with acute situations such as 'flu and infections as well as more long-term conditions, like arthritis and recurring complaints.

Naturopathy takes a distinct view of disease – placing importance on the individual's resistance and ability to overcome health difficulties, rather than on the nature of an infecting organism. 'It's the soil not the seed.' Have you ever noticed how some seeds never grow whilst others bloom and blossom, with the minimum of care. The quality of the growing medium is all important, and so it is with our own healthcare. When the body is operating under too much stress, or is under par, it is easy for the immune system to fail, and for things to start to go wrong. When you are feeling on top of things, and life is running smoothly, this is rarely the time that you succumb to opportunistic infections like colds and 'flu.

Symptoms are often seen as the body's attempt to increase elimination and to overcome the disease itself, or as signs pointing to the area of the real problem. A cold might well be a good sign of increased resilience on the part of the mucous membranes – particularly if it occurs after giving up smoking, for instance, when the body will need to expel a number of toxins that have accumulated in the lungs and bronchi. A skin complaint may point to a sluggish bowel condition; when the bowel is not functioning well, stresses are placed on the body's other eliminative routes – the kidneys, lungs, liver and skin. Skill is needed to determine whether the symptoms are a positive sign to be encouraged – a healing crisis, as distinct from a situation in need of support – a disease crisis.

After a full diagnosis has been made, the naturopath will draw on a wide variety of treatments to provide the best possible care in resolving the symptoms and improving the constitution. This usually entails some work on the part of the patient, who will need to be actively involved in their own healthcare. In aiming to give individuals the responsibility for their own health, the practitioner's role is most often as advisor – suggesting diets, providing herbs, initiating new lines of thought or exercise plans. Even the more physically based aspects of a treatment, e.g. an osteopathic adjustment, may require a commitment from the patient in terms of learning how to lift correctly or maintaining an easy posture, if the problem is not to recur. Often physical stretches or exercises will be recommended to carry on the good work from the treatment.

Once a course of treatment is underway, the naturopath may refer you to other therapists – a masseur for example; and continue as a co-ordinator or central focus for your ongoing health.

Most naturopaths will develop their own areas of specialization, so this is worth asking about at the initial consultation. Some may concentrate on the links between mind and body, focusing on an integrated view and being able to offer psychological counselling as a mainstay of the treatment. Others may rely more on constitutional change, using herbs, diet and hydrotherapy to maintain health.

Treatments usually last an hour, although some practitioners leave even longer for the first visit, or when using physical therapies. Courses of treatment vary in length, although most naturopaths will continue to fulfil a GP-type function; treating ongoing and changing health considerations as they occur.

Finding out more
Incorporated Society of British Naturopaths
Kingston
The Coach House
293 Gilmerton Road
Edinburgh EH16 5UQ
Tel: 0131 664 3435

Further Reading

Henry Lindlahr, *Natural Therapeutics*, C.W. Daniel Company
Ross Trattler ND DO, *Better Health through Natural Healing*, Thorsons.

NEURO-LINGUISTIC PROGRAMMING

Neuro-Linguistic Programming (NLP) is at the forefront of psychotherapeutics, gaining wide acclaim and offering a radically new way of interpreting our motivations and drives. The 'neuro' relates to the brain and the whole nervous system, and how we create our perception of the world; 'linguistic' refers to the words we say and the way we communicate with ourselves and others; and 'programming' emphasizes our ability to change, even at a most basic level. This set of tools builds together to form a way of acting effectively in the world, and of achieving change. A basic NLP tenet is that if you keep on doing what you have always done, you will keep on getting what you have always got.

NLP was born out of observations by Richard Bandler and John Grinder of the success of three therapists – Virginia Satir, a family therapist, Milton Erickson, a hypnotist, and Fritz Perls, the founder of Gestalt therapy (see Talking Therapies, pp. 305–6). They each used different styles of therapy, and were all extremely successful. The factors that were common to each of their practices were isolated and developed to form the basis for NLP.

These three therapists, and many others who were also studied, all appeared to operate from a set of pretty remarkable, and very useful presuppositions about life:

- every person is unique
- everyone makes the best possible choice available to them at the time
- there is no failure, only feedback
- every problem has a solution
- mind and body are part of the same system
- we already have all the resources we need. We need to develop access to these resources at appropriate times
- the meaning of any communication is in its effect – it is not what you intend to say, it is about the response and the experience of the listener (who may be yourself)
- If it is possible for someone, it is possible for me
- behind every behaviour is a positive intention
- the person with the most flexibility in thinking and behaviour has the best chance of succeeding.

Providing individuals and therapists with new insights into the differing frames of reference that we all use, NLP sessions are very practically based. The skills are used mainly as a tool for potentially dynamic personal change, and these techniques start by exploring the mode of thinking and feeling with which the individual feels most comfortable: some of us rely on visual memory, others rely on auditory memory, etc. (A kinaesthetic person might say 'that feels good'; an auditory person might say 'that rings true to me', and a visual person could say 'the picture looks bright'.) A hugely important area of communication is listening and giving feedback – 'I see' doesn't always mean that you have been heard. Assessments of eye movements, pupil size and direction of gaze also provide clues as to the importance of specific memories and where we store them – for instance as a personal reflection, something learned, or an inspired thought.

Ancient philosophy suggests that much dispute is born of mis-communication. Much human communication is non-verbal, and NLP provides many ways in which the communication between individuals, partners and groups may be identified, and offers techniques for making them more effective. They are easy to learn and put into practice, and most practitioners will include in their sessions instruction on those skills which are likely to be most useful. NLP techniques also work on our own inner communications.

Along with providing a useful way of managing change by offering ways to learn more about how effective we are and what motivates us, NLP techniques can be used very effectively for dealing with immediate issues. The techniques offer a variety of ways to diffuse stressful and traumatic memories by separating the feeling response from the picture of the event itself. This does not suppress the feelings, but it does allow them to be addressed more easily. In effect, what often happens is that if you are able to review a situation or event that occured without feeling the emotions that are connected to it, then your entire experience of that event changes, and the feelings also change to some degree. These techniques are often used by psychotherapists and counsellors to enhance the client's ability to look back at our emotional past and to learn from it.

NLP can also be applied to purely physically based responses, like allergic reactions, and can work to improve sports performance, as well as treating phobias and anxieties. Because it is so dramatically effective and has many commercial applications, NLP has become very popular in the business world.

For personal growth, health and problem solving, always consult a practitioner who has experience in that field. Sessions will vary in length and can be repeated as often as is needed. The work is all about learning how to effect change, so much of what is learned in a session will need to be put into practice, and this will often determine how much work, or how many appointments are made at any one time.

An area of research that is currently exciting many allo-pathic (or conventionally-trained) medical practitioners is psychoneuroimmunology. In the US they are investigating (and proving!) the connections between how we feel emotionally, and how our bodies work. They have been able to measure in a scientific way the changes that occur in the immune systems of individuals who have been exposed to emotional trauma or who are grieving. At this time, the reproduction of some specific cells which help rid the body of invaders, and also those which are involved in repressing tumour activity, is slowed down. The body's energy seems to be spent in another direction. Groups of individuals whose stress levels are high – for example, those facing the pressures of work deadlines, final exams, caring for sick or elderly relatives – have more sluggish immune systems which do not rise to the challenge of disease control as quickly or ably as those experiencing lower levels of stress.

It seems that when people feel emotionally depressed or are experiencing negative physical *or* emotional states, the way their bodies work is also depressed. This means that we can clearly see the link between our own thoughts, attitudes and beliefs, and the workings of the body. It seems that science has finally managed to prove that what we think can influence who we are and how we are – and that we can consciously choose health over disharmony.

It is being proposed that psychological factors are more influential in morbidity than smoking, obesity, blood pressure or exercise. The concept, for instance, that psychological stress may be as important a contributor to a smoker's health conditions as physiological stress is a radical one. I wonder if health warnings on cigarette packs might one day read: 'Warning – Stop and think WHY you are reaching for that cigarette'.

At least this is encouraging more people to recognize the integrity of the human individual – an entity comprising feelings and emotions that are intrinsic to a physical manifestation. Once again, we are seeing a branch of science prove the wisdom of natural healthcare. Once this connection is satisfactorily verified, perhaps allopathic medicine will do more to embrace a view of the human organism that is more than just a sum of disassociated parts.

The following exercises were devised by Maureen and Rob Lloyd-Owen of Poise. They will enable you to experience for yourself the effectiveness and ease of NLP. They are written just as they need to be spoken, so you can either read them on to a tape, or have a friend speak them for you.

Exercise 1
An inner journey to enliven your own health

This is designed to enable you to understand the power of metaphor to go beyond ordinary written language, and to put you in touch with the deeper meaning of your own inner thinking and feeling systems.

Read through the words in italics below, those enclosed between the two sets of double lines. Read through them carefully before you actually do the exercise. You could read the sequence on to a tape, or have a friend read the passage slowly to you, and then return the favour. Remember to pause when reading through the sequence. If it helps, talk it out loud to your friend, or tape your responses so that you can refer to them later. You may wish to repeat the exercise more than once.

1. *Go inside yourself, and allow an image or an idea to emerge when you consider the idea of what is 'natural'.* (Pause.)
2. *Really connect with this notion. Take a look at the idea or image. What do you see?* (Pause.)
3. *What do you hear – what sounds are present with the image?* (Pause.)

4. *What else can your senses feel, smell, taste? (Pause.)*
5. *Now silently repeat to yourself the word 'natural', while you are fully experiencing the image and all the feelings, sounds and sights associated with this word 'natural'. (Pause.)*
6. *Open your eyes, and review the experience, either make notes, review the tape you have made, or talk it over with your friend.*

Now you are going to repeat stages 1–6, but using a different idea:

7. *Go inside yourself and allow an image or an idea to energe when you consider the idea of 'wonderful health'. (Pause.)*
8. *Really connect with this notion. Take a look at the idea or image. What do you see? (Pause.)*
9. *What do you hear – what sounds are present with the image? (Pause.)*
10. *What else can your senses feel, smell, taste? (Pause.)*
11. *Now silently repeat to yourself the words 'wonderful health', while you are fully experiencing the image associated with these words. (Pause.)*
12. *Open your eyes, and review the experience, either make notes, review the tape you have made, or talk it over with your friend.*

Now comes an even more interesting task.
13. *Go inside yourself and say silently the word 'natural', and allow the image to come back with all the sights, sounds and feelings. (Pause.)*
14. *Whilst staying associated with the word 'natural', say*

silently to yourself the words 'wonderful health'.... and allow the image to come back with all the sights, sounds and feelings. (Pause.)

15. *Now, ask yourself what do I need to do to merge these two images, and to allow myself to have natural wonderful health. (Pause.)*

16. *Speak out what you see, hear, feel you need to do after you asked yourself the question. (Pause.)*

17. *Allow the images to merge, experience the wonderful sensations of natural wonderful health, and say silently to yourself while you enjoy those feelings: 'Natural Wonderful Health'.*

18. *Open your eyes and review the experience, either make notes, review the tape you have made, or talk it over with your friend.*

What do you need to change, if anything, in order to have Natural Wonderful Health?

Exercise 2
A circle of harmony to balance your whole being

This exercise will enable you to understand the power that you have to create resources for yourself which you can use whenever you need them. Do this exercise standing up.

Read through the words between the two sets of double lines below, as for Exercise 1. Read through the exercise carefully before you begin. You could read the sequence on to a tape, or have a friend read the passage to you, and then return the favour. Remember to pause when reading through the sequence. If it helps, talk your experience out loud to your friend, or tape what you say, or do both, so that you can relax into the exercise, and still be able to review your impressions later. You may wish to repeat the exercise more than once.

1. *Create a circle on the floor about two feet in front of you and three feet in diameter.*
2. *Recall a time when you felt whole, harmonious, and balanced, and when your health was excellent. If you cannot do this, make up a time, it is just as powerful.*
3. *Now see yourself in the circle as a whole, harmonious and balanced person, enjoying excellent health* (pause), *hear yourself talking and moving, and watch how you respond as a whole, harmonious and balanced person. Notice how good you feel about yourself as you watch this picture.* (Pause.)
4. *Now, move into the circle of harmony – into that picture of yourself where you are whole, harmonious and balanced, and access all of those resources again. See what you see, hear what you hear, feel what you feel.* (Pause.)
(Note: when talking aloud here, use the present tense 'I am' – be associated with all you see, feel and here.)
5. *Now remember that at any time in the future when you may need these resources they can be accessed by simply thinking of yourself in the circle of harmony.* (Pause.) *How does that feel?*
6. *How do you feel now?* (Pause.)
7. If these resources feel sufficient and you feel all right, you can stop – otherwise step out of the circle and repeat steps 2–6.

(Please note: this exercise can help you remember how you can feel, and also help you set goals for how you want to be.)

Finding out more
UK Training Centre for NLP
11 Buckland Crescent
London NW3
Tel: 0171 483 2384
Maureen and Rob Lloyd-Owen
Poise
Wyndcliff
17 Cowlersley Lane
Huddersfield HD4 5TY
Tel: 01484 460333

Further Reading

R. Bandler and J. Grinder, *Frogs into Princes*, Real People Press
James P. Carse, *Finite and Infinite Games*, Penguin
Change Your Mind and Keep the Change, Real People Press.

NUTRITION

Allergies • Organic Food

The foods we eat provide essential building blocks for continued good health. Nutritional advice forms a key element in all naturopathic work, and covers the range and types of food eaten each day as well as specific diets for individual purposes, for example, to treat a condition or to lose or put on weight.

We are what we eat – literally! Our bodies are constantly rebuilding, everything from our skin to our bones has its own cycle of growth and elimination, and the foods we eat provide the raw material for that growth. A good diet is one of the most important steps we can take towards continued good health and disease prevention throughout our lives, it is not just important for children and in convalescence.

There are many factors to consider when looking at the foods we eat – among others, their condition, the nutrients and benefits they can provide, how and when they are eaten, and their chemical components.

It seems obvious that our food should be in good condition – we would not choose to eat a rotting apple, or a piece of mouldy bread. We tend to tell a lot about the quality of a food from its appearance, and in the past this was a good indication of its state. Nowadays, however, this is often far from the truth. The many chemical processes that even fresh fruit and vegetables are exposed to is daunting, and this is before we think about processed, canned, or freeze-dried produce.

Much of the fruit we buy has been chemically grown and treated, waxed or even irradiated. The average apple has undergone 23 chemical processes by the time it reaches the shop shelves. Admittedly, some of these are repeat sprayings of fungicides, pesticides or fertilizers, but it still makes for a complicated chemical cocktail. So much for 'an apple a day ...'. It frightens me when I hear that the pesticides which are banned from our drinking water because of the health hazards they pose are the same pesticides that are routinely used on much of the food we eat.

Naturally or **organically grown foods** are the only viable alternative to slowly poisoning ourselves. On the whole they taste better, and the labelling is honest – when you buy an organic carrot, that's all you are getting: not a carrot plus an assortment of poisonous or noxious substances whose long-term effects on humans are unknown.

The market for organics is growing all the time. There are now more and more products available and the price is being lowered, although naturally grown produce is still much more expensive then chemically grown foods. A good variety of organically reared animals, milk and cheeses is appearing in the shops, along with a growing selection of fruits and vegetables. With careful shopping, up to 70 per cent of any diet can now be organic, and the difference will be felt straightaway.

How we handle food once it is in our hands is another

important consideration for ongoing health. The closer a food is to its natural state, the more beneficial it is likely to be. A large amount of raw food eaten each day ensures a good supply of nutrients and facilitates peristalsis – the way food is moved through the gut. Raw fruit and vegetables contain cellulose, a natural form of fibre which moves easily through the system cleansing it as it goes. The fresher the plant, the more vitamins and minerals it will contain. Vitamins fall into two categories – water soluble and fat soluble. The water-soluble vitamins are lost as soon as they are cooked, so even in winter raw foods form a valuable part of the diet.

The way that food is cooked can conserve or destroy its valuable nutrients. Steaming is better than boiling, for example, when the best part of the food is usually thrown down the sink with the water. Different cooking methods are more appropriate to certain seasons too: long, slow, oven cooking which conserves the goodness and energy of food is perfect for the winter months; quicker methods like stir frying seem in tune with nature as spring comes.

These are just some of the factors a naturopathic dietary therapist will consider when working out an individual eating plan with their patient. Obviously, personal likes and dislikes are important, but so too is recognizing that these are sometimes governed by the response of jaded taste buds, or by allergies. Our taste buds can adapt to large amounts of salt and chemical flavour enhancers, but once these are removed from the diet, they can revert to giving us a clear picture of the flavours and tastes we really enjoy.

Ordinary table salt should not, in fact, be on *any* table,

but moved to the bathroom. There is enough natural sodium in the foods we eat without adding extra to any cooked meal. In the West we use salt far too liberally as a flavour enhancer, and, like all flavour enhancers, our palates quickly adapt to want more and more of it. It is often added to cooking, as well as to prepared food, and is present in most tinned and processed foods. Once removed from the diet, the natural taste of food can shine through and the amazing recovery powers of your taste buds will delight you in their refound sensitivity. Too much salt added to the diet can lead to fluid retention and can compound high blood pressure and heart problems. Nature's own flavour enhancers, herbs and spices, are a much better all-round choice, and bring a host of nutritional and medicinal benefits with them.

Allergies pose a complicated challenge to naturopaths. Sometimes the foods we have an allergy to are those we crave, or that are a staple, regular part of daily meals. The connections between dairy intake (milk, cheese, butter) and mucous conditions is well documented – chestiness, sinus conditions and continuous cold-type symptoms respond well to the removal of dairy foods from the diet.

We still tend to think of cow's milk as a nutritious, health-giving drink: governments promote it and it is still provided in some schools. So many children's health concerns clear up when milk is removed from their diet, and it can easily be done. Substitute it with goat's or sheep's milk, or a plant-based milk like those made from soy beans or barley. Wheat has a proven implication in arthritic complaints, yet this too has a regular place in most diets. Where necessary, a practitioner may recommend abstinence from some everyday foods for a period of time.

Other allergies may be less obvious; I have an allergy to the oxylate family (tomatoes, rhubarb, spinach and sorrel are the main culprits) although sometimes just one member of a family can cause difficulties. The problems caused by an allergy can range from severe headaches to general low-energy feelings, or an aggravation of other conditions.

Genetic factors are important here, too – a growing number of Europeans are experiencing mild potato allergies, a direct legacy of the vegetable's prominent position in the diet over the last 100 years. Those with Mediterranean forebears may exhibit sensitivities to olives – they and their oil being widely used throughout the region. Or if a parent had a strong allergic response to a certain substance, then that may appear as a sensitivity in their child.

Allergies to the artificial additives and chemical compounds with which foods are adulterated are by far the most common.

Your naturopath will have two main concerns – to encourage a healthy and varied basic diet, and to deal with any specific health difficulties. They can suggest particular diets to help with a number of complaints, from arthritis to migraines, or may propose changes in diet from season to season.

Keeping a diet diary is a useful way of identifying any possible aggravations, and of getting an overview of our eating habits. You may be asked to keep one for a few days prior to your first visit and this, along with the information you give in the consultation, will help to build a clear picture of your current nutritional status. Many therapists will suggest a course of vitamin and/or mineral supplements for you to take, alongside the changes in your diet.

You may also be advised to add some foods – it's not all about taking foods away. The use of foods for their healing and curative qualities is another important aspect of naturopathy. Beetroot is a great liver tonic and can help with clearing the system; alfalfa stimulates and supports the spleen; cabbage is useful in cleansing the skin, and there are many other foods which support and help the body in similar ways.

I am currently seeing an increasing number of people who need to add some animal protein to their diets. Our disgraceful methods of animal production are encouraging more and more people to give up eating animal flesh altogether, some out of shame, and some with sound health concerns – flesh of this type is often seriously unhealthy for us. Some do very well, and are much healthier this way, but I believe that some people do need animal protein in their diet in order to stay healthy. It is also very important to ensure good dietary care when making a dramatic change like this, and a working knowledge of other protein sources is essential. Organic rearing and humane killing methods mean that dignity can be restored to the animals that we breed for human consumption, and to ourselves.

Dietary therapy is concerned not just with the foods themselves, but with the context in which they are eaten, the background, the season, and the condition of the foods themselves. All these factors are as important as the individual's constitutional needs. Life-style makes a difference, as does a person's inherent vitality and their ability to eliminate unwanted substances from the body. Whether their circulation is good, if they have a sedentary job, at what time of year they feel their best and a variety of other factors will all help to determine individual requirements.

Treatment is often an ongoing process, with sessions increasing in regularity as health considerations change. Most often, an initial course of appointments will be followed up by visits at the change of each season, and then an annual check-up.

There are also dietary therapists or nutritional counsellors who do not have a naturopathic training. They work independently, and their main areas of expertise will tend to be the nutritional values of the foods. These therapists often rely on supplementing the diet with vitamins, minerals and other formulations to achieve fuller health.

Keeping a diet diary is a brilliant way to gain a host of insights into the way you eat, as well as what you eat, and when. Keep one faithfully for a week, making an entry every time you eat, or drink, rather than leaving it till the end of the day. Be sure to note what type of food you are eating, e.g. whether it is a home-cooked, or ready bought meal, and the situation, e.g. if you are grabbing a snack while at your desk, or settling down to dinner with friends.

Diet analysis sheet

Day :

Breakfast: Drinks:

Lunch: Snacks:

Dinner:

Physical feelings after eating:

Overall energy levels:

Emotions:

Notes:
Keeping a diet diary can both highlight possible allergens and indicate how balanced your basic diet is. Review it at the end of the week, and you should be able to spot some clear patterns in terms of what you have eaten, and why. This may be enough in itself to spur you into making any changes, and building on your strengths

Finding out more
Incorporated Society of British Naturopaths
Kingston
The Coach House
293 Gilmerton Road
Edinburgh EH16 5UQ
Tel: 0131 664 3435
Nutrition Society
10 Cambridge Court
210 Shepherds Bush Road
London W6 7NJ
Tel: 0171 602 0228
Green Farm Nutrition Centre
Burwash Common
East Sussex TN19 7LX
Eating Disorders Association
Sackville Place
 44-48 Magdalen Place
Norwich NR3 1JE
Tel: 01603 621414

Further Reading

Manuela Dunn Mascetti and Arunima Borthwick, *Food for the Soul*, Newleaf
Kirsten Hartvig ND and Dr Nic Rowley, *You are What You Eat*, Piatkus
Ross Trattler ND DO, *Better Health Through Natural Healing*, Thorsons.

OSTEOPATHY AND CHIROPRACTIC

Osteopathy is an important aspect of naturopathy, adding a major corrective physical therapy to the simple philosophies of nature cure. Devised by an American, Andrew Taylor Still, in 1874, it is a method of directly addressing structural difficulties in the body, and influencing the whole of the body as a result. Forms of physical manipulation have been used for centuries, as seen in ancient Native American hieroglyphs, forming part of Hippocrates' teachings, and even impressing Captain Cook in the 1700s during his travels to Tahiti.

Osteopaths assess the integrity of the spine and the rest of the body using a structural, mechanical model. The spine is comprised of a number of separate bones linked together to provide a solid protection for the spinal cord. There are seven bones or vertebrae in the neck, or cervical region, twelve in the upper and mid-back (thoracic area), and five in the lower back (lumbar spine) before reaching the sacrum and coccyx, or tail bone. The size and shape of the bones varies from one region to another, and the joints between all these differently-shaped bones are designed to enable full movement in a range of different directions. (The direction of movement changes from one area to another.)

Obviously, problems can occur if there is bad posture or incorrect body use, when the muscles can place stress on these joints, or if there is any sudden exertion or an accident, such as a fall or whiplash injury. Lifting something too heavy, or staying in a taxing position for too long, can cause back pain, as can not getting enough support from a bed that is too soft, or from badly-shaped seating. As well as addressing any problem in the back, an osteopath will assess the effects on other parts of the body, and can also treat a range of complaints from frozen shoulder to housemaid's knee, tennis elbow and flat feet.

The presence of asymmetry – e.g. protecting an injury, or compensating for an area of weakness, can set up a chain of imbalance throughout the body. This may stress some areas more than they are designed to deal with, and cause a problem with secondary aches and pains. An obvious example of this is if you hurt your leg or foot, and continue trying to get around. Limping can put pressure on your lower back, and cause pain and discomfort in both hips, or throw your spine off-balance, generating pain higher up.

The integrity of the spine is also vital to full health because in the vicinity of each vertebral joint is the space through which the nerves leave the protection of the spinal cord to travel to the various organs and areas of the body. These nerves carry the stimuli which enable the body to work, and also relay messages back to the brain.

If there is irritation or dysfunction in this key area, then the messages relayed by the nerves may become impaired, and the areas of the body they feed may not continue to work optimally. For this reason, most treatments will include an assessment of the spine, whether patients are suffering with poor digestion or breathing difficulties, as well as more obvious concerns like headaches.

Osteopaths assess the structural integrity of the spine and the other joints of the body by observing movement restrictions and areas of immobility, and through palpation or touch.

After your history has been given, and the details of any specific complaint you may have, the practitioner will ask you to undress as far as your underwear to allow a proper look at your back. Some practitioners will provide gowns, like those you will find at a hospital, which are open down the back.

First of all you will be asked to carry out a range of active movements with the osteopath watching you closely – like walking up and down, bending, and turning your head. You will then be taken through a range of passive movements (these require no muscular effort, rather the practitioner will move your body for you).

A number of neurological tests and an assessment of muscle condition will follow, and the practitioner will then investigate the degree of movement between each separate vertebra. This is done by placing a light hand pressure on each one in turn, whilst moving or mobilising those on either side of it.

This takes place with the patient either seated or lying down, and should cause no pain, although some slight discomfort may be felt if the osteopath finds an area with a problem. At this stage a diagnosis can be made, and the treatment may stop while the osteopath informs the patient of their findings, and explains what is to happen next.

If the practitioner has found an area of displacement (often called a lesion) they are likely to manipulate it back into position. To do this, the body is used as a long lever, with a specific vertebra at the fulcrum. This may entail some careful twisting, or putting the body into strange positions to set up the manipulation, which is carried out speedily and, usually, painlessly. Sometimes the manipulation will involve a thrust directly on to the site of the pain or difficulty, without moving the body as a whole. When this takes place a clunk or click sound may be heard, usually accompanied by feelings of instant relief. When the vertebrae in the neck are manipulated, this clunking sound appears to be much louder, but it is not at all dangerous.

The osteopath may make a number of manipulations in different areas of the body during a treatment, and may also demonstrate specific exercises to maintain mobility throughout the area, or to strengthen certain muscles groups that are important to the maintenance of good posture. These are often given as homework, and need to be repeated as prescribed, and will be followed up in subsequent sessions.

Obviously, there are some people who should not be manipulated in such a way, and some health concerns preclude this form of treatment. Post-menopausal women, who are at risk of osteoporosis (thinning of the bones), those with a history of tuberculosis and anyone in acute pain are a few examples. An osteopath will determine what form of treatment is advisable when they take the case history.

Nowadays, osteopathy is often practised as a specialty in its own right, and a number of osteopaths are not naturopaths.

The first appointment will usually last for an hour, if the practitioner is also a naturopath, or 30–45 minutes if not. Subsequent visits vary from 20 minutes to an hour, and may need to be at weekly intervals until some improvement is seen. They may then be reduced to monthly visits, then an annual check.

Another form of manipulative therapy is Chiropractic. This is the main choice in north America, and is becoming more popular throughout Europe. Chiropractors work in a very similar way to osteopaths with a few important distinctions. They rely almost exclusively on x-rays for diagnosis, whereas osteopaths tend to use them as a back-up measure to confirm any findings. These can be taken quickly because many chiropractors will have x-ray equipment in their practice. The benefits of this thorough approach need to be balanced against such exposure to radiation, however. Because chiropractors spend much less time actually examining the patient, some appointments can be completed in ten minutes.

The other main difference is in the style of manipulation. Chiropractors tend to prefer more direct thrusts, while osteopaths prefer 'long-lever' techniques. There is much debate as to which is easier for the patient, but an important point is that neither is likely to cause any degree of pain or tissue damage. Direct thrusts involve place pressure on the vertebrae, and using a quick, specific push to reposition it. Long-lever techniques involve positioning the body so that the vertebra in question is encouraged to right itself, and will require minimal force from the practitioner to complete the repositioning.

A branch of Chiropractic has recently evolved called McTimmoney Technique. This concentrates on a more wide-spread approach to manipulation, incorporating some of the best Chiropractic techniques with osteopathic concepts to develop a form of bodywork which is gentle on the body.

Osteopaths can now be found at a few hospitals, where their treatments are available on the National Health Service. These are pilot schemes, and as yet the government has no plans to extend their availability. Both osteopaths and chiropractors work at natural health clinics and in private practise, and some also advertise in the yellow pages. There are fewer McTimmoney practitioners, because the therapy is still relatively new.

The following exercise is a particularly good one for strengthening and stretching the back and neck, and will also give the lymphatic system a boost.

Sit upright on a chair with both feet flat on the floor. Slowly begin to lower your chin down on to your chest, and raise your arms to interlock your fingers just behind the crown of your head. Gently lower your hands on to your head and let their weight bring your head down lower. Slowly relax the arms and your elbows will move down and towards each other in front of you; the weight of your arms drawing your head down still further. You should be able to feel this stretch in your neck and upper back; but if you are not generally active, or if there are any areas of immobility in your spine, you may feel the stretch right down to your sacrum or tail bone.

Hold this position for ten to twenty breaths, and then very slowly reverse the process; slowly lifting your elbows and raising your hands, and then last of all, your head.

Next, let your head move slowly backwards, making sure that your back stays straight. Do not stretch your head back, just let it reach the point where you begin to feel the muscles at the front of your neck start to tighten. Jut your chin up and out past your upper teeth, and feel the stretch down into your sternum or chest bone.

Hold this position for ten to twenty breaths, and then slowly lift your head back up to an upright position.

First aid in cases of back pain is straightforward. Stop whatever you are doing, and get into the rescue position (see below), to relieve any pressure on your spine. Consider the use of an ice-pack directly on the site of the pain - use a packet of frozen peas or corn, and apply to the area for five minutes, repeating every twenty minutes.

The back care rescue position entails you lying flat on your back with a pile of cushions in front of your bottom, raising your thighs directly up, and letting your calves lie flat on top of them. One of the easiest ways to achieve this is by lying on the floor with your bottom up against the sofa or a chair. Remain in this position for as long as possible, or until help is sought.

Finding out more:
Natural Therapeutic and Osteopathic Society
14 Marford Road
Wheathampstead
Herts AL4 8AS
Tel: 0158283 3950
British Osteopathic Association
8–19 Boston Place
London NW1 6QH
Tel: 0171 262 5250
British Chiropractic Association
Premier House
Greycoat Place
London SW1P 1SB
Tel: 0171 222 8866
Institute of Pure Chiropractic
(exponents of the McTimmoney Method)
14 Park End Street
Oxford OH1 IHH
Irish Osteopathic Association
17 Windsor Terrace
Portobello
Dublin 8
Tel: 01 473 0828

Further Reading

Susan Moore, *Chiropractic*, Optima
Stephen Sandler, *Osteopathy*, Optima
Peta Sneddon and Paolo Coseschi, *Healing with Osteopathy*,
Gill & Macmillan.

OUTDOOR CONTACT

As we become more insulated against the elements in our sturdy homes and hectic lifestyles, it becomes ever easier to lose contact with nature, even though the natural world still governs our lives through the seasons, the daily cycle of light and dark, and the growth of all living things.

Our bodies and emotions are still tuned to a natural clock; influenced by the seasons and in need of contact with the elements. (See Cycles and Seasons, pp. 77–82.) After a day spent indoors, we'll often use the need for fresh air as an excuse to go for a short walk, or to stand in the garden for a while. Yet opening a window would provide the fresh air. What we really feel we need, and often do not know how to express because it is such an instinctive drive, is contact with 'the great outdoors' – to move freely and see nature, perhaps walk on some soil, feel the wind move us, or the sun's touch, or to gaze at the stars. We become unhealthy in body and spirit if deprived of such contact for long.

Many a gardener can tell of the magic of working with soil, and of feeling close to other growing things. There is an amazing sensation to be had walking barefoot on clean grass – you can really feel in touch with the planet with which we live.

227

I once read that if topsoil were the equivalent of our protective layer of skin, then grass would be the hair of the giant organism, earth. This image has stayed with me and, although very romantic, it is an amazing thought to be caressing the earth's tresses every time we reach down and touch a patch of grass.

When sunlight touches the skin we can produce vitamin D – essential for health. When we are in natural surroundings, particularly in the presence of moving water, we are bathed in life-enhancing negative ions. It is hard to resist the Native American teachings that we are all part of the Great Spirit – ourselves and all living things, and Grandmother Earth and Grandfather Sky.

The quality of the air we breathe is so important. We need fresh, clean air for our lungs so that oxygen can be carried by the blood to every area of the body. Every cell has its own cycle of renewal – it breaks down and is then rebuilt according to its innate sense of timing. Oxygen is an important building block in this process, and the construction of healthy, non-malignant cells relies on oxygen, amongst other things, being available in the right amount. When the air we breathe is polluted, instead of large amounts of oxygen, we provide our bodies with lead, carbon monoxide and a whole host of other noxious and dangerous substances.

As our lungs become polluted they are less able to achieve the important energy exchange which is necessary to prevent a build-up of carbon dioxide in the system. The lungs play a vital role as one of the body's main routes of elimination, and any under-functioning here places increased pressure on the rest of the body.

In cities throughout the world, incidences of breathing difficulties and lung disorders increase in line with elevated air-pollution levels. Asthma and a wide cross section of allergic reactions and minor immune system dysfunctions occur with increasing regularity as we continue to damage the quality of our air.

Trees are the answer for they increase the oxygen content of air faster and more efficiently than anything else. Sadly, as we destroy the rain forests and other woodland areas across the world, we point towards our own destruction. On a more local level, tree-lined avenues, parks and woodlands are really the only places to take exercise or walks.

The ability to breathe fresh, clean air is a basic human need. When we exercise, one of the purposes is to increase the amount of oxygen we take in. It isn't necessary to take large gulps of fresh air – just breathing normally should supply all the oxygen you need, and the simplest of activities will speed up your intake.

Walking is one of the best all-round exercises you can do; it is a gentle workout for the whole body, exercising most muscles and improving abdominal tone. Walking gradually increases your oxygen needs and your lung capacity, thereby improving general fitness. Increasing oxygen requirements whilst walking along busy roads, or in other heavily polluted areas simply increases the rate of poisoning you will experience.

A regular intake of fresh air is a necessary part of all-round good health, and it is vital that this air is clean and good. Many of us live in towns and cities, or close to the motorways which criss-cross much of the countryside, or to industrial centres. All these situations create a special need for fresh air, and it is well worth searching out areas that will provide this.

This issue is vital and many people, once they have started to enjoy the pleasures of more outdoor contact, feel that they have a responsibility to campaign in some way for anti-pollution legislation, local clean-air campaigns, rain forest preservation or whatever will make a difference, and leave our air pure and fit to breathe, and the rest of our environment safe and clean.

Many therapies and health philosophies recognize the importance of outdoor contact for our continued good health, and both Ayurvedic medicine and traditional Chinese medicine, along with naturopathy, emphasize the importance of balancing the elements within us.

Our bodies are a part of nature, and are made from the same building blocks that we see around us. We can say that we have the energies of fire, earth, air and water within us, as well as around us, and we can work with those elements to achieve balance and health. As natural creatures, when we reinforce our connections with the world of nature, we support and encourage all our own natural functions.

Spending time with nature enables us to strengthen a part of ourselves, and bringing the elements of the natural world to play in our daily lives enriches us in many ways. It is here that we learn about the passage of time, death and rebirth, and our own cyclic nature. We watch as the delicate balance between order and chaos shifts and moves, creating natural patterns that show us the beauty of creation. The dimensions of space and shape combine in landscapes and visions that please the heart and the eye.

Addressing the balance of the elements is a powerful way to effect our own healing. If you think about life on this planet, it exists in the way that it does because of the balance of the elements. If the sun were to shine more strongly, and the place was only a few degrees hotter, our lives would be completely different. If there was 20 per cent more water, we would all be living in the seas! Changes to our internal elements can also have an immense effect upon our way of living.

Fire

When we look at the sun, we see our inspiration and source of illumination.

We can see for ourselves how well balanced our inner fire is by asking a few personal questions:

- How enthusiastic and joyful am I?
- How well do I allow the spark of spirit to manifest in my life?
- Do I welcome spontaneity and change?
- Do I get enough actual sunlight in my life?
- Are my physical symptoms showing an excess of heat (red skin rashes) or an absence of heat (cold all the time)?

Balance your inner fire by spending some time every day following your heart, and allowing your natural joy to surface. Learn to avoid excesses in all areas of your life from feelings to appetite, and keep your body temperature even, never getting too hot or too cold. Make space for your spiritual life, and allow it to manifest in your life, and keep your body fuelled by eating well and regularly. The body's digestive fire, like the

---

sun, reaches a peak at mid-day, and it is good to follow this rhythm and eat the main meal of the day when the appetite is greatest. Acknowledge your sexual and creative energies and find appropriate means of expression. Take some time to be out in the sunlight each day.

Earth

The earth is mother to our physical body. It is the world we live in, therefore representing the body, and it is a powerful agent of transformation, just like ourselves. It is the element that most keenly shows us the changes in weather and season; freezing over in the winter, burgeoning forth with new growth in the spring and summer, and cloaking itself in the gold and browns of autumn. It is concerned with our nurturing and our nourishment, and in the body it is most keenly represented by the stomach and spleen.

Ask yourself some of these questions to see how well integrated the earth element is for you:

• How in touch with my body do I feel?
• How do I nourish and nurture myself ?
• Can I trust my body to transform things?
• Am I in the right situation in which to flourish?
• Do I spend time in contact with the earth?
• Are my physical symptoms showing an excess of earth (overweight, heavy), or a deficiency (underweight, rare appetite)?

Work towards balancing this element in your life by having

regular contact with the earth – through gardening, potting, or by regularly playing with the soil and sand. Make sure that you nourish yourself well, and eat plenty of yellow foods like corn, squashes, pumpkin and apricots. Nurture yourself by making time to spend with yourself, and by doing things that bring you pleasure and comfort. Regularly take time to stop and rest, and get in touch with your inner self. Develop opportunities for relationships and friendships where you can both give and receive warmth and love. Experience for yourself the rich abundance of life, and how it may make you feel satisfied and complete. Pay attention to your physical home, your body, and its needs and pleasures, and also to your other homes – the place where you live, and the local area, and the environment of the planet – make yourself feel 'at home' all the time.

Air

Air is all around us all the time. It is here, right now, going up your nose, and touching your skin, and it is also on the other side of the world blowing clouds around. It is a strange mixture of something that is immediately necessary for us, and something that we often feel quite distant from. Breathing fresh, clean air is essential to life, yet it is invisible and most times goes unnoticed and forgotten. Air can represent our thoughts, which appear and disappear just as quickly as a breeze and are equally invisible. In the body the lungs have the greatest connection with air, but the skin can be in contact with it all the time as well.

The answers to these questions will shed light on the element of air in your life:

- How clear are my thoughts?
- Can I work well with new ideas?
- Am I an effective communicator?
- Do things move freely through my life?
- Is it easy to welcome new things and to let go of what no longer serves me?
- Can I think of any physical or mental symptoms that relate to this element, e.g. flatulence, indigestion, difficulty of moving things through the body, inability to think clearly?

Encourage the element of air in your life by allowing yourself to be impulsive and mercurial sometimes. Air is light and fast and brings new possibilities and beginnings with it. Air is the ability to change ourselves in a flash – once we recognize that it can be done. Air carries the messages of spirit, and can be everywhere all at once, so allow it to breeze into and around your life every day. Make contact with air – walking and being outdoors and playing – with a kite, or a windmill, or just through going out on a windy day. Respect the tremendous power of the winds and honour them by letting them sweep through your life on occasion, blowing away any unwanted clutter and leaving your world spring-like and fresh. Delight in the excitement that you can experience when this happens, and allow yourself to feel light and free.

Water

Water represents the feelings and emotions, and our own way in life. It has a phenomenal range of qualities, from the perfect compactness of a raindrop, to the raging power of a waterfall and the vastness of the sea. It has tremendous versatility, being able to hew its way through the strongest materials, and yet soft and gentle enough to bathe in. It is essentially fluid and mobile, but can freeze over into the hardest substance, or boil and bubble and embrace chaotic movement. It is a symbol of cleansing, and of change. In the body water is represented by the bladder and the kidneys, but all parts of the body contain some water, and it is the element that is present in the largest amount within us. This is what responds on such a large scale to the pull of the moon as it moves through its monthly cycles.

Ask yourself these questions to explore the element of water in your life.

- How in touch with my emotions am I?
- Do I allow time for my feelings?
- Am I aware of my own courage and strength?
- Does the world around me reflect my own inner beauty?
- Is there time for stillness in my day?
- Do I have any physical or emotional symptoms that are water-related – crying a lot, bloating, watery discharge, great thirst or dry and flaky skin?

Balance the water element in your life by ensuring that you are aware of your abilities and your potential. Review your connectedness with the fluidity and strength of water, and allow yourself to feel like a drop in the ocean. Make time to express your feelings and further creative endeavours with certainty. Cultivate your own inner strength and wisdom, and maintain your physical flexibility and fluidity. Consider meditation as a way to contact your own inner stillness and the richness of your inner world. Make regular visits to the sea, lakes,

> rivers and other water features. Allow yourself to trust in your own way, even though it may seem willowy or uncertain, and recognize the power that lies within water.

Finding out more
Friends of the Earth
26–28 Underwood Street
London N1 7JQ
Tel: 0181 490 1555
Greenpeace
30–31 Islington Green
London N1 8XE
Tel: 0181 351 5100

Further Reading

Dylana Accolla with Peter Yates L.Ac, *Back to Balance*, Newleaf

Lynn V. Andrews, *Flight of the Seventh Moon*, Arkana

Jonathon Porritt, *Seeing Green*, Blackwell

Patrick Whitefield, *How to Make a Forest Garden*, Permanent Publications.

PERSONAL PHILOSOPHY

The development and nurturing of a positive personal philosophy is an important facet of total healthcare. We unconsciously strive to make our lives fit our own idea of how they should be, and the body is the most immediate physical thing we can mould to fit our desired image. It is immaterial whether this philosophy is purely in relation to health or more all-embracing; whether it is an individual perspective or shared with a large group. What is important is to have a clear idea of your own purpose, and an understanding of how your life works. With this understanding, goal setting, decision making, good health and general life management are all made possible.

Taking responsibility for your own health is an important adult skill. Any philosophy which absolves the individual of this responsibility in my opinion cheats them out of their own growth. Taking responsibility means integrating healthcare into your lifestyle in a beneficial way and taking full possession of your body, the physical reality of who you are.

In our early history, health difficulties beyond the individual's own care would be taken to the local medicine man or woman, a healer or Shaman. This magic person achieved their healing through involving their patient in a truly holistic approach. Special plants, herbs or potions might be given, but a major part of 'the cure' was the dynamic quest or ritual in which the patient would immerse themselves. This meant that the psychological and spiritual aspects of the person were wholly focused on cleansing and healing their own body. They were totally involved in their own transformation. That these methods were completely and utterly successful is borne out by our presence here right now.

While I am writing this I am reminded of a recent television programme about giving birth. One of the prospective fathers, on expressing his feelings about the coming birth, said: 'I don't know how it works at the hospital – whether they let fathers stay for the birth, and whether they'll let (my partner) move around in the early stages.' He didn't know whether 'the professionals' would allow this woman to move freely if she felt that was what she wanted. Who has responsibility here?

In the last century, particularly during the growth in power of the medical profession, we have all been encouraged to dissociate from our bodies, to hand over any defective bits to a professional until they can be cured and returned. As a society we desperately need to reclaim our integrity as individuals and recognize our own potential expertise in our own specialist subject – ourselves. Only when we see our bodies as ourselves, as the place where we live, will we be able to claim good health; good all-round health – physical, mental, emotional and spiritual.

Check out your own attitude – what happens when you get a headache or stomach pain? Do you curse the inconvenience and try to remove the problem as you would a stain from a piece of fabric – or do you stop and ask why this is happening. Has your diet been at fault, your stress level too high, have you been ignoring your body's need for rest? And what do you do? Do you take a pain-killer, so that you can stop feeling what is wrong; or do you seek to resolve what is wrong in the knowledge that if you find and treat the cause of the discomfort then the pain will naturally disappear?

Obviously, allopathic, or conventional medical treatments have their place – surgery really is the only life-saving answer that we know about for a ruptured appendix (although the incidence of inflamed and ruptured appendix is significantly lower in those eating whole food diets), but this way is just another philosophy. We are educated to regard it as the norm, in fact it is one way of looking at healthcare, and it seems to be a pretty faulty one. The health service is failing now partly because its premise is incorrect. Suppressing symptoms without recourse to their cause is not health, it is a recipe for degenerative disease and mounting illness during old age.

As a mainstay of our hierarchical society, the health service continues the myth of personal powerlessness. There are strong connections between society as a whole and its institutions. Religious dogmas often seem far removed from the spirituality of their original teachings; and attempts to embrace the individual in social welfare can erode individual rights. Rather than individual free-dom, the corner stone of hierarchy seems to be the removal of personal choice.

Reality is a fact. How we experience it is absolutely up

to us – if you imagine reality as a landscape, every philosophy will give you a map or grid to superimpose on the landscape in an effort to make it more understandable. We all use grids or maps, and a conscious knowledge of our own grid (or philosophy) allows us to make sense of our journey.

The more informed we become, the more equipped we are to make choices. In relation to our personal health and welfare, this may mean looking beyond society's main offerings to redefine how our needs may be met. This is an enormous challenge, particularly for those of us who have lived our lives within the security of a narrower outlook. If we believe in the value of our own growth, facing this challenge provides us with a valuable opportunity to take part in our own development; to measure our own nurturing, and to participate fully in our own process of transformation. This is full health – our ability to respond and change and move in order to stay alive.

Further Reading

Neil Freer, *Breaking the God Spell*, Falcon Press
Ivan Illich, *Medical Nemesis*, Pelican
David Watkins, *Urban Permaculture*, Permanent Publications
Anne Wilson Schaef, *When Society Becomes an Addict*, Harper and Row.

QUIET

Mention quiet, particularly to a city-dweller, and a whole host of words spring to mind – peaceful, silence, golden, renewal, relaxation...

We are exposed to almost constant auditory stimulus, sometimes chosen, sometimes not; e.g. other people's radios, in-store music and traffic noise. When we hear something, it impresses us, makes our mind work to understand, or classify, or make choices about it. I was once appalled to discover, on taking a holiday in a small seaside village, that it took days to clear my head of an assortment of song lyrics, ditties from commercials, hack-neyed phrases, and background buzz – all the things that fill my head without my even realizing it.

Finding a quiet time each day is important, whether we use it to clear our minds, or for more formal reflection or meditation. Without this, our own inner thoughts risk becoming lost in the mêlée of incoming sounds and ideas. Uninvited noise can also be a great irritant, adding to our stress levels and robbing us of the opportunity to relax.

The effects of this type of stress are insidious – we often don't realize how much noise we have tolerated until we quite suddenly notice a silence. Even welcome sounds like music can dull our senses if they become continuous; we can also then become inured to their beauty and less discerning. While we are unconsciously concentrating on blocking out background noises, our bodies can suffer; breathing becomes shallow, and there is less available energy for necessary tasks like digestion and repair work.

We all need time alone with our own thoughts and ideas in order to appreciate our own values and validate our beliefs. One wonders at the possibility of original thought while we are constantly bombarded with other people's ideas and society's values, tastes and instructions.

During pregnancy, loud noises and the physical effects of continually resisting low-level noise can cross the placenta. If it troubles the mother, then it can trouble the foetus at a time when it should be allowed to continue its growth uninterrupted. The extremely positive side of this is that parents and others can talk to the unborn baby during the last stages of pregnancy.

A quiet time can be one of the most valuable periods of the day, both mentally and physically. Sharing silence with others is a profoundly effective way of improving true communication. We have become very 'sound-reliant'. When we rely on verbal communication it is easy to forget other vital methods of expression. The unspoken communication between lovers and friends is tremendously important and gives us the opportunity to reflect on how we normally convey our thoughts, ideas and feelings. Our body language and the 'vibes' we give off can convey our feelings very well – sometimes very much more clearly than the words we use.

Some of our talk is also necessary only in order to avoid

silence, which can make some people feel awkward or vulnerable, so talk and noise are a protection. It is in silent times that we can heal ourselves; make conscious our inner motivations, and bring creative notions and ideas to fruition. Our selves can be very good company, and if we make friends with ourselves then the quiet times can become rich with the cementing of that relationship.

Some religious houses and other communities offer the opportunity of silent retreats; a time to experience this solitary adventure alone, or with others. Some may structure the retreats by marking the beginning and the end with some form of ritual, ceremony, or inspirational readings. These can set the tone of the retreat by suggesting a focus, or by unifying the group.

Other cultures such as the Native American spiritual tradition use this as an important part of their personal growth, and a regular part of daily life. The experience of turning inwards in this way, particularly in the company of others, can be remarkably liberating. A personal silent retreat can be the perfect way to get in touch with our own inner selves, and deserves a regular place in every busy schedule. Those same feelings of uninterrupted communion with ourselves can be experienced in any quiet moments we can find.

Finding out more
The Right to Peace and Quiet Campaign
PO Box 968
London SE2 0RL
National Retreat Association
24, South Audley Street
London W1
Tel: 0171 493 3534

REFLEXOLOGY AND METAMORPHIC TECHNIQUE

Barefoot therapy has a prominent place in natural health-care. We all know how much good feeling can be generated from this small but important area of the body – simply freeing your feet from shoes and stockings or socks at the end of the day can bring relief to most people. Letting your feet breathe unhampered by synthetic fibres or the confinement of footwear has important health applications too.

Many foot problems stem from lack of air, or from mis-shapen shoes. Fungal complaints like athlete's foot thrive in moist, warm conditions, and allowing feet to breathe is an important part of avoiding this type of complaint. People often find that the natural shape of their feet bears little resemblance to the shape of the shoes that house them for up to eighteen hours each day, so it is little wonder when corns, bunions and areas of hard skin develop. You can check this for yourself with two sheets of paper and a pen: stand with one foot on a sheet of paper, and your weight distributed evenly on both legs. Bend down and draw around the shape of your foot, or have someone do it for you. Now put on your shoes, and repeat the process, comparing the results. The differences are usually most striking with women who wear high-heeled shoes.

Taking early morning dew walks on a patch of clean grass or sand, paddling in the cool, clear waters of a stream on a hot day, or amongst the waves along a beach, can bring enormous pleasure. It also directly stimulates this important part of our bodies, and through them, every other part of ourselves. Learning to explore things with your feet, discovering textures and defining shapes are all very worthwhile activities. We spend so much time using them to bear our weight that we can easily forget just how sensitive our feet are.

There are people with disabilities who write, paint, and do much more with their feet. I knew a woman who trained her toes to move up and down independently of one another, and thought she was quite remarkable in this, until told of another woman who had done the same, then another – it seems all it takes is time and concentration! It seems only right that this capable, sensitive and useful part of the body should be given lots of care. Bringing feet into contact with fresh air and walking barefoot for some time each day allows the muscles of the foot to be exercised, and it is very grounding; putting us back in touch with the world we walk on. I feel, too, that this warms some distant genetic memory in the tremendous feelings of well-being that it can generate. Our distant forebears spent much of their time barefoot, only using a protective covering when needed.

In many groups and societies today footwear is removed as a sign of respect, at times of personal reflection, and as a sensible health measure. A growing number of people do not wear shoes at home, giving their feet some

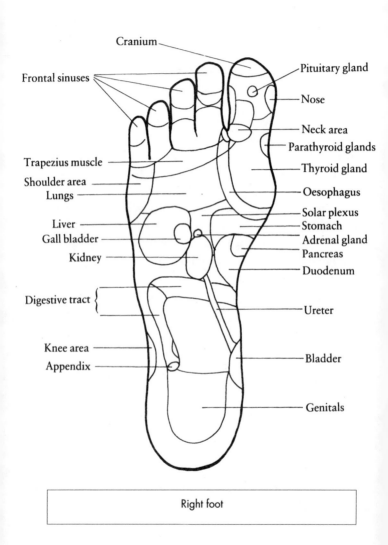

Right foot

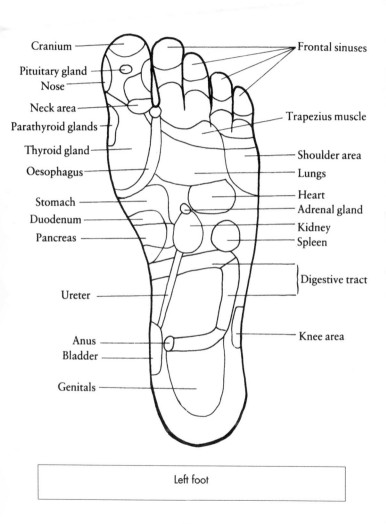

Left foot

freedom, and keeping the dirt of the streets out of the house. This can also help mark the transition from the end of the working day, or of outdoor pursuits to time at home.

In our search for health and well-being, we cannot ignore the promise and the joy that being good to our feet can provide. There are two therapies that treat the whole body through direct contact with the feet: reflexology and metamorphic technique.

Reflexology seeks to treat all parts of the body through the reflexes in the feet. With the client seated, or lying back with their head raised, the Reflexologist works using tiny pressure movements over both surfaces of the bare foot, and around the ankle. The movements follow a map which details parts of the body and its corresponding point on each foot.

The spine reflex, for example, runs all the way along the inside of the foot from the heel to the top of the big toe; and the solar plexus point is just below the ball of the foot in line with the second toe. The liver, spleen and other organs are all represented, along with general areas of the body like the head and neck (represented by the toes).

Reflexologists aim to effect changes to general health, as well as to stimulate specific areas, or to relieve tensions in particular spots. They develop a sense in their hands which enables them to feel areas that are in need of work, through the changing textures of the feet. Although this is a very pleasant experience in the main, the client may well be able to feel that some spots are more sensitive than others, or to notice connections with other body parts – e.g. experiencing stomach gurgles while the digestive

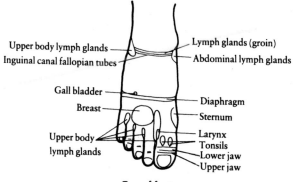

Upper body lymph glands
Inguinal canal fallopian tubes
Gall bladder
Breast
Upper body
lymph glands

Lymph glands (groin)
Abdominal lymph glands
Diaphragm
Sternum
Larynx
Tonsils
Lower jaw
Upper jaw

Top of foot

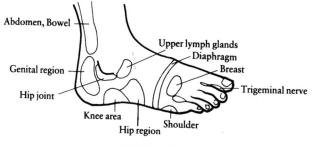

Abdomen, Bowel
Genital region
Hip joint

Upper lymph glands
Diaphragm
Breast
Trigeminal nerve

Knee area
Hip region
Shoulder

Outside of foot

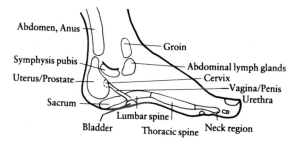

Abdomen, Anus
Symphysis pubis
Uterus/Prostate
Sacrum
Bladder

Groin
Abdominal lymph glands
Cervix
Vagina/Penis
Urethra
Lumbar spine
Thoracic spine
Neck region

Inside of foot

system is being worked on or relaxing more deeply while the area relating to the solar plexus is covered. An experienced practitioner will notice the changes in a client over subsequent treatments and be able to chart their progress.

Some people love their feet being touched or massaged, and respond very well to it, but even those who are a little anxious soon find reflexology to be very settling and relaxing. The practitioner's touch should be just firm enough not to tickle, but not so hard that it is ever really painful. Occasionally certain areas will be a bit sensitive, and this is taken to be a sign of some form of imbalance in that region.

Reflexologists usually recommend a short course of treatments – perhaps four or six, to see how well you get on with each other and with the therapy. Follow-up visits can then be six months or one year apart.

Metamorphic technique takes quite a different approach. Using a light, feathery touch, practitioners concentrate more on the emotional level of the client. They maintain that the foot represents the nine-month gestation period in which all of our mental, physical, emotional and spiritual patterns are set. The events which regulated our mother's changing hormone levels are maintained to mark our growth and establish our future patterns and responses. By gently smoothing out the areas of the foot where these are found (often represented by hard skin, changes in texture or structure), the behaviours or stresses that can lead to ill health are relieved.

Although working at such a level, the technique is not at all interactive – the practitioner is quite likely to be talking about unrelated topics or the theory of metamorphic technique rather than whatever they are perceiving with their hands. My own feeling is that change can most beneficially and truly occur with conscious participation, but there is no denying that positive sensations and good feelings are generated in the treatments, and that changes can be seen after just one session.

This is also a very gentle and non-threatening form of treatment, which can be employed alongside other treatments like massage therapy or counselling, or as an introduction to some form of physical contact. In the spirit of wholeness, though, it is the responsibility of the practitioner to share with their patient or client whatever insights may have been gained. Not to garner such information, or to withold it, seems strange. Sessions usually last about thirty minutes, and may include a similar form of gentle work on both hands, and on the head. It is usually left for the client to decide on the number and frequency of repeat visits.

Gentle foot massage will generate pleasant feelings throughout the body. Knowledge of the reflexology foot charts can encourage you to cover all areas of the foot, and although it will not be the same as a reflexology treatment, it will make you feel good. It is a good idea to massage your feet in some way every day. This can easily and simply be done in the bath or shower, by taking a few minutes to carefully lather and clean each foot. Alternatively, use a little warmed olive or sesame seed oil to lubricate your hands, and simply stroke each foot several times while it is still warm from the water.

A five-minute massage at the end of the day can help relaxation and aid restful sleep. Warm the oil, sit down and take your time to make sure that you work gently over the whole area. Start by using soft strokes that run the length of your foot from the heel towards the tops of your toes. Develop this by using small circular movements that press a little more deeply into the softness of your feet. Work your way over each foot in turn, and finish by simply holding and warming each foot between the palms of your hand.

Add a metamorphic-type massage after this, by gently running the index and middle finger of one hand along the inside edge of your foot from right behind your heel all the way along to your big toe. Make several gentle, sweeping movements along this edge using a light, passing touch that feels like a gentle breeze. Then follow the same line making tiny, light circles all the way along the length of the foot.

Sharing massage like this is a wonderful way to deepen communication between lovers, friends, and family members. Giving a foot massage is easy if you have learned how and practised on yourself, and receiving one is even more relaxing than doing it yourself.

Finding out more
British Reflexology Association
Monks Orchard
Whitbourne
Worcestershire, WR6 5RB
Tel: 01886 21207

British School of Reflexology
92, Sheering Road
Old Harlow
Essex CM17 0JW
Tel: 01297 29060

Irish Reflexologists Institute
3 Blackglen Court
Lambs Cross
Sandyford
Dublin 18
Tel: 01 295 2238

Metamorphic Association
New Cross Natural Therapy Centre
67 Ritherdon Road
London SW17 8QE
Tel: 0181 672 5951

Further Reading

Anya Gore, *Reflexology*, Optima
Avi Grinberg, *Holistic Reflexology*, Thorsons
Rosalind Oxenford, *Healing with Reflexology*, Gill & Macmillan
Gaston Saint-Pierre and Debbie Boater, *The Metamorphic Technique*, Element Books.

RELAXATION

With all the pressures in our hectic lives, we need to find time to relax, unwind, and rejuvenate ourselves. Taking time off from busy schedules and switching off the mind is not always easy, but there is a huge range of relaxation skills and techniques that can work very well, once we make the time for them, and give a commitment to ourselves to try them. Some can be practised in any ten-minute gap during the day, others require more of an investment in time, but all yield remarkable results. There is also a range of videos, tapes and books to guide you through the available techniques. Simply sitting in front of the television, or reading a book is not necessarily relaxing – this can be a skill that we need to learn, and one that we deserve to spend time on.

Relaxation is only possible if we feel safe and secure in our chosen environment. Physical comfort is important – we need to feel free from the restrictions of tight clothing, and to be comfortable and warm. Some people, usually those with excess energy, will find it most easy to relax whilst expending that energy physically, so a brisk walk may be the best choice for them. Or that may be a preliminary to any quieter work. Most often, though, full relaxation is a sedentary practice.

When we are stressed, it is more than a feeling of being under pressure – are bodies are affected too. Our system will be full of adrenalin, giving that 'all psyched-up' sensation. This is great if we need to meet an immediate crisis, but when sustained for hours, days or months can lead to nervous irritation and physical exhaustion. This can lead us to further confuse our bodies by taking artificial stimulants like caffeine, and this load is compounded by suffering aggravation from an assortment of pollutants. General worries and concerns, unresolved issues and the ups and downs of our emotional responses add to the stress.

Removing all of these difficulties would be a pretty tall order, but just letting go of our concerns and switching off that ever-ready attitude can be remarkably soothing. It's rather like preparing an elaborate meal – there may be several pots simmering on the stove and a dish in the oven, but it's still necessary to leave the kitchen for a while, even if only to set the table. We may well never get our lives 'just right' or completely stress-free, but perhaps the most useful skill we can cultivate is the ability to switch off from it all and allow ourselves the experience of relaxation and renewal.

Our minds are absolutely capable of juggling a number of projects, and we rarely switch off our consciousness altogether. This time-off is as essential to our total well-being as any other element of our balanced lives, like periods of leisure, and play. Perhaps the most important function of relaxation is in providing a time for the body and mind to fully unite and heal.

When a muscle is tense it cannot function properly – neither receiving an adequate blood supply with all the essential nutrients which that brings, nor getting rid of its waste products. Without these functions, the mechanism of muscle contraction can begin to fail altogether.

A primary concern of most relaxation techniques is to still and quieten the body. This can be achieved in a number of ways, and the simplest is by bringing the areas of tension to our conscious awareness in order that we might then issue the mental instruction to relax. Among the formalized relaxation techniques are biofeedback, autogenic training and others which all concentrate primarily on the physical response – it is not easy to relax while a big part of you is tense. There is equipment that can help you recognize tension in the muscles, and there is a variety of tricks to still the conscious mind. If relaxation therapy is a new idea for you, you may like to begin with the simple techniques described later in this section. There are also relaxation therapists who will be proficient in a number of different techniques to aid relaxation, and relaxation classes are held at many libraries, civic centres and natural health clinics. Here a group of people can go and, sitting in comfort, be talked through the techniques together.

Many people believe in starting at the other end – with meditation or mental focusing exercises, but the aim is always the same; to still and unify the body and mind. If stress is not a chronic problem, there are many everyday pursuits which can aid relaxation including taking holidays, listening to music, becoming engrossed in some creative pursuit or hobby, breathing deeply, walking, dancing, and, of course, simply being quiet. The comfort of another's touch can be deeply soothing and relaxing, and in this less than tactile world, something we can often miss out on. We can tend to perceive touch as being mainly sexual or familial, but there is a tremendous love to be received and given between friends and partners; simple hugs and physical gestures can make us feel comfortable and easy in ourselves.

One of the most immediate ways to aid relaxation and feel better generally is with the aid of **relaxed breathing.** So often when we feel tense or unaware, our breathing can become shallow and insufficient. Remembering to simply stop and take a few deep breaths can be a useful short-term fix. Learning relaxed breathing is a way to ensure long-term benefits.

Sit in a comfortable chair with your back quite straight, or if you prefer you can learn this while lying down. Place your right hand flat on your upper chest, in the middle just below your neck. Take a few normal breaths, and you will probably find that this hand is moved up and down by the air that is filling your upper lungs. Now place your left hand flat on your belly, just covering your belly button.

Take a long, slow, deep breath in, and aim for it to reach right down to your left hand. Imagine the fresh breath of air filling your lungs from the bottom up, and filling your whole upper body with inspiration. Feel your rib cage open and expand as fresh air fills up the sides of your lungs, then let this huge breath out. Feel your entire torso gently contract as it relaxes back into place. Start taking more deep, regular breaths, right down into this place where your left hand is resting. If you look down, you will see it slowly rise and fall as the air inside your body pushes it out. Your right hand, held high up on your chest, should remain still.

This can feel a little strained at first, but you will soon find that it is not in fact tiring, but relaxing and rejeuvenating. Practise for ten minutes, twice a day, and you will notice that breathing this way becomes easier, and more relaxing. Remember to stop for a moment and take a deep relaxed breath if you feel yourself becoming stressed or tense. You should find that you can adopt this as your normal way of breathing quite quickly, and you will feel the benefits in all sorts of ways. Breathing this way gives the organs an internal massage, and it also improves peristalsis (the way food is moved through your system).

Sit in a comfortable chair, with your spine straight, and your feet flat on the floor. Make sure that you will not be disturbed. Loosen any tight clothing, and slip off your shoes. Close your eyes for a moment and see what picture will come to mind when you think of relaxation, comfort and ease. It may be something like an image of you sinking into a comfortable arm-chair, or standing in the sun and feeling its warmth reach deep into you. See if there is a way to use the image, or a symbol of it in your relaxation – you might choose the symbol of the sun, or of a cushion, for example.

1. Adjust your seat, and make sure you are quite comfort-able. Take a deep breath in, and close your eyes. Start with the little toe on your left foot. As you breathe in, move your awareness to that spot, and see the image of relaxation that

you are using there. Say to yourself 'relax' as you breathe out, and move on to your next toe. If you do not have a strong image of your own, use the image of a light going out, or of being touched with a feather. Continue to breathe in and out, concentrating on the image as you inhale, and silently saying 'Relax' as you breathe out. Work your way through each toe, and then on to the ball of your foot, your arch, up over your instep, around your heel and then up towards your ankle. Take your time, and keep your breathing easy and regular.

2. When you have finished relaxing your foot, move on up your leg, making sure to relax every part of it from your ankle, up your shin, your calf, all around your knee, and all of your thigh, including your hamstrings at the back, and the inside and outside. Repeat this whole process with your right leg, starting with your little toe on your right foot, and working all the way up to the top of your thigh using easy, relaxed breaths. Then work your way up your trunk, starting with your buttocks, and reaching round to include your pelvis, extending up either side of your spine, and around your ribcage, until you reach your shoulders. Keep planting your image of relaxation, and using your breath to let go of any tensions while you silently repeat the word 'relax'.

3. Relax your way down first your left arm, and then your right, going all the way down to the tips of the fingers on each hand. Then come back to your neck and relax each side of it, all the way up to your scalp, working in short chunks and keeping your breathing easy and relaxed. Relax your scalp, and your hair, and pay particular attention to your hairline, and the area close to your temples and around your ears. Take your time, there is no rush – this is perhaps the first time you will

have experienced such total body coverage, and such a complete relaxation, so do not hurry it. Relax your brow, your eyelids, all over your face, including those tight jaw muscles, and then down to the tip of your nose.

4. Take a deep breath, and imagine yourself settling back into your body, finding it looser and more relaxed, and allowing you more movement and freedom. Find a place to settle where you feel yourself to be truly centred in your body, and take a few deep, easy breaths from this place.

When you are ready, take a deep breath in, and as you breathe out, slowly open your eyes. Now take another deep breath in, and as you breathe out, gently stretch any part of you that feels the need to move. You will have been sitting still for a while now, and although relaxed, you may feel that your legs or your arms or your spine would appreciate a stretch. Take your time and appreciate the feelings that you are experiencing. Do not rush to get up, and when you do so, keep your movements slow and steady for a few minutes while you readjust.

Practise this once a day, spending however long it takes to get from the tips of your toes, to the tip of your nose, and then deep inside yourself.

Further Reading

Jane Madders, *Stress and Relaxation*, Optima
Louis Proto, *Total Relaxation: The Alpha Plan*, Penguin.

SELF-ANALYSIS

Analysis is a term many of us are familiar with. Strictly speaking it refers to psychoanalysis, a distinct form of therapy that is based on the teachings of Freud, or analytical psychology which is based on the teachings of Jung. The work of analysis is based on a detailed and ruthless exploration, within a highly formalized structure, of the client's (or analysand's) history of events and emotions from birth to the present day. Freud's teachings were based on his own personal experiences and those of the people who consulted him in his private practice. He believed that early conflicts were at the root of most individual distress, and did much pioneering work in the field of human sexuality. The fundamental belief in Freudian analysis is that a person's psyche is completely determined by the events in the first five years of life. Expressions that have fallen into common usage such as penis envy and Freudian slip stem from here. He maintained that most women are traumatized to some degree by the discovery that they they do not have a penis, and that our true, or deeper, feelings can often spring to the surface seemingly by accident, but really to speak our own truth. Jung expanded on these early ideas and focused more upon the concept of archetypes or universal images and the positive effects of consciousness, or conscious awareness, and the commonality of our experience.

Entering analysis requires a strong commitment, as well as a real need, and can involve up to five sessions each week for many years. Many analysts prefer the client to lie on a couch during the session, and will sit out of their line of vision. This has given rise to the expression 'doing the couch trip'. Analysis is not to be considered or undertaken lightly; it is a profound choice that is likely to affect every area of one's life. As the name implies, it involves sorting through and analysing all the events, thoughts, feelings and happenings of everyday life, as well as earlier, more ingrained and deeper or older beliefs and experiences. The techniques used are varied, but all focus on bringing remembered events into the light of consciousness, where they may be thought through and reviewed and then put together to form a clearer picture of one's life.

Many of the techniques used within analysis can be used alone, forming a type of self-analysis. This is something that is free and available to everyone who chooses it. This useful tool is rather like an exercise in de-coding. Often, the real relevance or significance of occurrences in our lives, and our own information about these events, seem to be clouded from consciousness, or expressed only through symbols in our feeling world, or in our dreams.

We can all, for example, learn to understand our dreams (and something of our lives) by interpreting the symbols that we use in them. You don't need to be a Shaman, or a clairvoyant to build your own vocabulary of symbols. Just as once you learn the meaning of a word, that is the word you use to express an idea or to identify something, so symbols are simply non-verbal words, and once learned (or interpreted) will be used in the same way. Part of the magnificence of symbols is that they will convey not just one word at a time, but a whole story.

Thinking about symbols and what they mean to you is a good place to start in **understanding your own silent vocabulary**. If you accept that they may be more than they seem, then this exercise will be of benefit.

Make some time when you can sit quietly and still, and get in touch with your own silent self. Some people do this best through meditation (see pp. 188–91) or you may find that simply relaxing will do the trick. Make sure that you will not be disturbed, and will be able to settle down to this gentle, inner work.

Choose a range of symbols and images that you remember from your day-dreams, fantasies, or night-time dreaming. You may like to prepare a list beforehand, and can spend some time drawing this up. The symbols can be as simple or elaborate as you choose, and include some elements of the natural world:

- a tulip
- a landscape
- an ocean
- a tree
- the sun
- a blade of grass
- the night sky ...

263

Now, close your eyes, and imagine a blank screen in front of your eyes. Reach forward and switch it on. One by one, place the images you have chosen to explore onto the screen in front of you, and see what happens. You may find that the image evokes feelings and emotions, or sensations within your body, or that it stirs memories of past events, or that it changes and becomes like a film as it tells a story in front of your eyes. Stop, switch off the screen, and record your findings.

Develop this, now, into a slightly different format. Keep your screen blank, and think about a range of ideas, or concepts, or feelings, and see what appears on the screen in front of you. You might think of 'home' and see what appears – perhaps it will be a country cottage with roses around the door and smoke curling out of the chimney, and drifting across the twilit sky. Does it feel as cosy as it looks? If so, perhaps this is an image or symbol of security. Insecurity might be portrayed as the cottage at night-time, with no lights and being ravaged by a storm, or by its complete opposite – a grey, city tower block or an industrial unit. Work through whatever range of feelings and ideas you choose, then, when you are ready, stop, switch off the screen and record your findings.

This is a wonderful way to begin a dialogue with your inner self, and you may find that you can use this silent screen technique for gaining understanding of other aspects of your self. You will discover that your own silent vocabulary is a wonderfully rich and self-renewing source of wisdom for you, which is full of worthwhile surprises and is totally unique.

Analysing dreams is an effective way to keep tabs on our own feelings. Keeping a **dream diary** is a lovely way to honour the unspoken communication we have within ourselves, and interpreting those dreams cements the relationship between our consciousness and what seems to be going on underneath the surface.

Make a clear decision to start recording your dreams, and mull the idea over for a few days. Prepare for the project by choosing a book or pad in which to note down what you remember of your dreaming, and placing it by your bed. Choose a pencil to write with, and place this with the pad. Before you go to sleep, think about the idea of remembering your dreams, and see yourself in your mind's eye writing in your dream book the minute that you wake. As soon as you wake up, reach for your dream diary and write down everything that you remember. Initially it may be only a little, or some disassociated images, or perhaps just a feeling. Start to build up a trust with yourself by making an entry of whatever you remember in your dream diary every morning, and you will soon find it becomes a valuable piece of material.

Some people go back to their dream diary later in the day, and review the connections between their dreaming and their waking lives. Or you may like to write on only one side of the page, and leave the other side blank for a drawing, or for noting any comments or realizations that come to mind later. Let your inner feelings be your guide, and choose a way that is right for you.

Analysis of our conscious actions and motivations can often be made easier by distancing ourselves from them. Simple measures such as writing down the situation that is in need of clarification in a letter and posting it to yourself can be remarkably revealing. Listing the pros and cons of any decision can also yield unexpected results, and important insights. One patient of mine agonized for weeks about whether to move house. She eventually made a list of all the reasons why she should, all the benefits to be gained, and all her objections. She found herself with two pages full of good reasons to move, and six reasons not to. One of the six was the immensely powerful 'I don't want to.' She was able then to see the decision in a much clearer light – as being between what made logical sense but betrayed her feelings, and what she didn't want to do, but might be seen as a good idea. She had loaded down the logical side because, for her, one ounce of feeling equalled at least three pounds of logic in any equation. She chose not to move.

The psychic and healer Betty Balcombe uses a triangle to help clarify situations. Draw a triangle on a sheet of paper and write your current challenge in the centre. On the left of the triangle list the events which led to the dilemma, track right back to when and where the difficulty began. On the right side, list what needs to be done, what help is needed, who needs to be consulted or what extra information is needed. This gives you a clear picture of the past, the present, and what action can be taken. When all the possible action has been dealt with, the choices become much clearer.

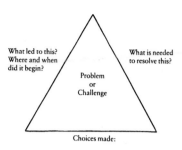

Self-analysis could also be called self-regulation or self-understanding, and can lead to a more complete and holistic understanding of ourselves and our actions. It enables us to use more of our mental capacity, and to integrate it with the rest of our experience.

Finding out more
Association of Jungian Analysts
5 Eton Avenue
London NW3
Tel: 0171 794 8711
Society of Analytical Psychology
1 Daleham Gardens
London NW3 5BY
Tel: 0171 435 7696

Further Reading

Betty Balcombe, *As I see It*, Piatkus
Eric Berne MD, *A Layman's Guide to Psychiatry and Psychoanalysis*, Penguin
Dr Brian Roet, *All In the Mind?*, Optima.

SELF-EXPRESSION

Art • Drama • Music • Voice • Dance • Toning

This is an essential part of living life to the full. We have a number of different drives, desires and urges to express, and keeping things in is rarely good for us. If you assess the balance of your life right now, you may well find that it is loaded in favour of work and rest. Few of us make time for our playfulness, creativity, sensuality, in order to develop our communication skills, mental alertness, physical prowess and sense of self. Society, along with our religious, cultural, gender and other stereotypes imposes its own pressures. Our roles tend to be fairly tightly described, and often there is little room for, or acceptance of, our own need for balance. Sometimes there just isn't the time to show strong feelings and emotions, to be vulnerable or very strong, to exhibit leadership skills and other powerful qualities.

We need to let the poet within ourselves express itself, whether through words, writing, movement, imagination, or through exhibiting a sense of excellence and elegance in all that we undertake. Whenever we create in this way, we act as transformers – moving energy from one aspect of our lives into another, and this can have a profound effect on the way we think, the way we act, and how our body works. Expressing creatively can aid us in problem solving and mental agility, it can also shift physical blocks and allow us greater emotional satisfaction.

There are many creative forms that can have therapeutic applications. Art, drama, play and dance therapy, amongst others, can form part of a supportive everyday routine. There are professional practitioners for all of these subjects if you feel in need of some structure and encouragement, and they can all certainly yield benefits when experienced on your own. Any sort of creative pursuit can be a fulfilling part of our lives. We all have creative energy, and it is there to be used. The variety of channels for this is enormous – some people pour it into their work, others separate it completely. Whichever you choose, it is important to acknowledge its role in your life as a fundamental part of living life to the full. Whether you express that creative energy biologically through bearing children; professionally, in the choice of a career in the creative fields; in your leisure time, or in your very private life is a matter of personal choice. You don't need to join a group to express your creativity – drawing or painting your feelings, or putting them into dance is something you can do at home or wherever you are; when the mood takes you or as part of your daily schedule. Drama and play are not ostensibly solitary pursuits, although if you have ever watched children at play, totally immersed in a private imagining, you have an idea of what is possible. On this level, the adult alternative would be constructive fantasy. Taking some time each day or at least each week to enrich your creative talents while leaving aside any work ethic can be wonderfully beneficial. Letting go of the need to be in control, or to behave in a certain, specified way is incredibly liberating, and can be lots of fun too.

Drama therapy or **psychodrama** is a popular choice of creative pursuit with a therapeutic bent. It takes place in groups of anything up to thirty people (although around twelve is usually the norm), and involves the other participants who act out the roles of characters in your own life, and then you in turn may play the part of someone important to them. Under the direction of the therapist, this allows the opportunity not only to figure out individual situations in an active and realistic way, it also draws on the intuition and feelings of the other group members. A variety of resolutions to any theme can be explored and experienced, and this dynamic form of acting out can quickly lead to an understanding of what feels right. Sometimes our true feelings can become buried underneath the obligations and restrictions that come to bear in real life situations, and this opportunity for make-believe can yield tremendous insights. After each enactment, time is given to reflection on the true feelings that emerged. An intimacy and feelings of safety are soon generated by groups that work in this way, and to aid these, the meetings may start with the therapist suggesting some group games. These are most often mental and physical exercises aimed at increasing the trust between group members, and act as a gentle warming-up period for the work to follow. Most people find these very enjoyable, and just as beneficial as what happens in the rest of the class.

Art therapy seeks to explore and release feelings through their expression in drawing, painting or modelling. These can then be interpreted using the artist's own symbology and/or the insights of the therapist. This direct means of expression by-passes the cognitive or censoring part of the brain and can reveal valuable clues as to the artist's own self, as well as providing an exciting new way to tackle involved or difficult matters. Art therapy can be explored on its own, or as part of many psychotherapeutic models. Or, you can do it yourself, without analyzing it, for the great pleasure it can provide. Although often taking place in groups, art therapists will also offer individual sessions. Many people find the group situations offer more security, especially if they are not experienced with this medium of expression – it is sometimes difficult to get started and having other people around can relieve any pressure. This is also a 'safer' place to start – allowing time to feel easier with this way of expressing yourself before exploring it more deeply. The contribution and insights of the other group members can also be extremely helpful. Different classes will take a variety of approaches; some using the time to focus on a theme which can then be illustrated; others using the class time in a more analytical way, by discussing homework for example.

Music as therapy is used a lot by people with mental and physical disability, providing a valuable means of expression and stimulus. Its use has become more widespread to meet the universal need for new avenues of expression and ways to understand the inner feelings that we have and which are sometimes difficult to validate. Pouring emotion into music is what makes it good – allowing it to resonate with something within the listener. The mood-changing effects of music are known to us all. Its evocative nature marks it out as an effective means of communication, and it has many uses within the community, unifying groups and creating atmospheres more effectively than just about any other measure. Gentle, soft sounds and easy melodies can aid relaxation and meditation; faster, more rhythmic music can help with more energetic activities. Using music as therapy may be the perfect way to begin to develop creativity, or a safe form of channelling emotions, or an energetic release. There are many ways to work with music – concentrating on rhythm and its hypnotic effects, for example, as in drumming, or on performance. Most usually, this therapeutic use of music is active, involving playing an instrument or singing, although it may also involve listening to music. People are often surprised to find how well they can evoke a feeling with an instrument. If someone were asked to play a violin, their initial reaction is likely to be refusal. Being asked to be *LOUD* on a violin, however, presents few problems. Once you feel this confidence, it becomes easier to let the feelings through, and from there comes the ability to acknowledge and begin to understand and accept them.

Using one's voice can be a wonderfully healing experience. Whether it is through singing, or chanting, or toning (see below) the feeling of 'playing one's own instrument' is deeply rewarding. A perfect method for creative expression, singing can teach us much about our own abilities and motivations and help us with our own flow of energy throughout the body. So many people think that they can't sing or hold a tune, and while a performance singer requires special training, learning to express oneself through the voice can unblock massive creative potential for personal growth on many levels. Music and **voice therapy** are usually conducted (!) in groups, although most therapists also offer individual sessions where deeper, more analytical work can take place.

Dance has always been an important part of human experience – as a means of personal expression, for connecting with the environment, bonding within the community, and as ritual. Dance therapy encourages individuals to explore their body through movement. Various styles have developed; some concentrating on the therapeutic aspects of what our body positions and movements say about our inner feelings; others focusing on the development of creative expression and freeing our own inner patterns and rhythms. Working in groups, sometimes with music sometimes not, the dancers can allow their bodies to flow and move in a free, unstructured way. The teacher may point out areas of restricted movement by mirroring them, or by inviting the dancer to find words or another way of demonstrating the feeling behind their action. Classes usually begin with some warming-up exercises before going on to expand individual movement sections. This is a wonderful choice of therapy for those wanting to get more in touch with themselves physically, and also for those who feel that they intellectualize too much. Moving freely and expressing our feelings through our bodies is something we all knew how to do in childhood, and dance is an excellent way of recapturing that childlike sense of freedom. There is real magic to be experienced when you give yourself to the dance, and a sense of wonder the first time your body moves knowingly, without conscious planning. The physical work-out involved in a class and experiencing the freedom to move creatively, strengthens the links between mind and body. This can have spin-offs – one being the wonderful side-effect of encouraging greater flexibility in a variety of other areas of life. Participants often experience the benefits of classes overflowing into their everyday lives. Once a confidence is gained, it becomes easier to express creativity and physicality in other ways and in a host of other situations.

One of the simplest forms of self-expression is through the use of voice. You know already that it can convey a multitude of different feelings, emotions and messages through its tone, as much as by what you say. **Toning** is a wonderful way to free up your body and your voice, and to learn some of your body's own intonation and subtle harmony. It is a simple technique to learn, and to put into practice, and is one of the most richly rewarding voice techniques that I teach. All sounds have vibrations, and the sounds we make ourselves will move and vibrate through the body. Certain sounds have an affinity with different body parts, and with different states of harmony and well-being. Toning is a way of identifying the sounds that your body needs to make and hear, and shows you how to use and clear those sounds in order to help resolve blocks and conflicts, not just in your body, but in other areas of your life.

Try this exercise for yourself right now, and you will begin to get a feel for how **toning** can work for you:

Sit comfortably, close your eyes, and take a few deep, easy breaths. Centre and still yourself so that you feel quite settled. Now take quite a deep breath in, and sing 'la' out. Choose any note, and don't mind if the note changes, just sing to the end of your breath. Straight away, breathe in again, and repeat the 'la', again with any note that comes. You may find that the notes change, or alter their clarity quite spontaneously. Some of your notes will sound clear and sweet, others might be huskier, or throaty, or sound weaker or tinny. Keep the rhythm of breathing in, and singing out 'la', and do not worry too much about understanding or analyzing this now. You may find that you quite naturally repeat certain notes, and if this is what you are inclined to do, then work with it by focusing on those sounds, and repeating them until they become clearer. If you notice that the note changes within each breath, then follow that. Let the sound lead you where it needs to.

This exercise is quite invigorating, so you may start to tire after a few minutes. That is fine. Relax, and return to it another day. If you do not naturally stop after about ten minutes, start to wind it down. After each toning session you should find yourself feeling refreshed and energized. Do this daily, and let your own voice lead you to developing this further for yourself.

Finding out more
Open Centre
188 Old Street
London EC1V 9BP
Tel: 0181 549 9583

Laban School for Movement and Dance
Goldsmiths College
Laurie Grove
London SE14
Tel: 0181 692 4070

Dance Education and Training
5 Tavistock Place
London WC1
Tel: 0171 388 5770

Person-Centred Art Therapy Centre
17 Cranborne Gardens
London NW11 0HN
Tel: 0181 455 8570

Playspace
Short Course Unit, Polytechnic of Central London
35 Marylebone Road
London NW1 5LS
Tel: 0171 486 5811 ext. 465

Playworld
2 Melrose Gardens
New Malden,
Surrey
Tel: 0181 949 5498

Living Art Training
11 Stowe Road
Ravenscourt Park
London W12 8QB
Tel: 0181 749 0874

Dancing on the Path
39A Glengarry Road
London SE22
Tel: 0181 693 6953
Irish Association of Drama, Art and Music Therapists
PO Box 4176
Dublin 1

Further Reading

H. Blatner, *Acting In*, Springer
T. Dalley, *Art as Therapy*, Routledge & Kegan Paul
J. Fox, *The Essential Moreno (dramatherapy)*, Springer
P. Holmes and M Karp, *Psychodrama: Inspiration and Technique*, Routledge
Keith Johnstone, *Impro (Improvisation and the Theatre)*, Methuen.

SHIATSU

All matter is composed of energy, and there is a range of therapies that work with the energy of an individual as it manifests in and around the body. There are many different approaches to this work, and healers work with this energy in a variety of ways. (See Healing, pp. 118–23)

Shiatsu practitioners follow a system of energy channels in the body corresponding to the acupuncture meridians. They apply a constant pressure to points they call tsubos which cover the whole body. This pressure is usually applied with the fingers and hands, directly onto the skin, although the practitioner's feet and elbows can be used on heavier parts of the body like the hamstrings muscles at the back of the legs. Most usually, the practitioner begins by deciding whether there is an overall condition of insufficient energy (kyo) or unexpressed energy (jitsu), and the treatment will vary according to this judgement; either dispersing any pent-up energy, or helping the body to conserve it. Some practitioners will take the pulses, or use tongue or facial diagnosis to help reach this important decision, while others rely on their psychic or intuitive skill and experience. Once the body has begun to balance generally, more attention can be paid to specific points along the particular meridians or pathways that the practitioner senses are in need of attention. The pressure used in Shiatsu usually feels very positive, although sometimes it may build up just to the point of pain. An experienced practitioner will be able to read the body well enough never to exceed this point.

Shiatsu originated in Japan and is still used there, and in China, as a form of primary healthcare, regular treatments being seen to be an active preventative measure. Dependent upon your individual needs, you may expect to feel either deeply relaxed or pleasantly energized after a treatment. Sessions usually last for about one hour, with the initial consultation lasting longer to enable a health history and other important information to be exchanged. As this sort of work is so energy reliant, it will vary considerably between individual practitioners, and it is important to find one with whom you feel a good energetic connection.

There is a charming story of a man in Japan who tried to find somebody to give him Shiatsu. He 'phoned for a visiting practitioner, and settled down to await his arrival. The Shiatsu Master who usually ran this service was unable to attend him, and a recently qualified student of his went along instead. So, the newly qualified practitioner arrived, and began his work. After only a minute, the man stopped him, saying 'I asked for shiatsu, not a student'. Despite the visitor's assurances that his qualifications were indeed sound, the man explained that: 'Your hands are busy – that is no way to give Shiatsu.'

This illustrates the quality of the work involved – the person giving the Shiatsu treatment must have 'empty hands' – hands that are totally receptive and responsive to the body on which they are working. The perfect training for this is in a refinement or cousin of Shiatsu, called **Jin Shen Do**. Many people maintain that whether the work they chose to pursue is actively physical, as in shiatsu, or subtler in nature, as in Jin Shen Do and similar disciplines, the understanding and ability to sense that is cultivated in these other practices is a prerequisite for beginning treatments.

Jin Shen Do practitioners use a similar map to those who practise Shiatsu, but rarely use pressure on the tsubos or body points, preferring a holding or slightly pulling touch. This is altogether different from a Shiatsu treatment, feeling much less physical, and seeming to reach a deeper level within the individual. More time may be spent on diagnosing a person's condition, and again this may be through light touch or psychic assessment, and the practitioner will then seek to encourage the flow of energy through the body with these gentle contacts. The whole body is not usually covered in the same way as in Shiatsu; rather the Jin Shen Do practitioner will select a smaller number of points and hold each for a longer period of time. This form of treatment has been likened to the ancient Chinese 'Art of Listening', in that work is done in a meditative state and the feeling afterwards is that one's body, with all its silent stories, has been truly heard.

Both forms of treatment require the patient to be at least partly undressed, and although Jin Shen Do may be performed with the patient lying on a couch, the more active Shiatsu usually takes place on the floor. As part of a session may involve use of the practitioner's full weight on the patient's body, a wide floor space is required. This usually consists of a thin, padded mattress similar to a futon which is then covered, so that the body is fully supported.

Treatments with both these therapies usually take place with the patient lying down, so that they may be as relaxed as possible. The work can be carried out however the patient is placed, but while lying down they will be comfortable and can feel quite secure – it is easier to to close one's eyes and therefore relax more fully in this position. It also allows the practitioner an easy contact with most of the patient's body, an important point because nothing is less conducive to relaxation than to have somebody fumbling to reach the inside of your arm, or having to move you around too much.

Most treatments take place in a reflective or meditative atmosphere, and there is no rush. As important as the treatment itself, is the time taken immediately afterwards to reflect on what has occurred, and to reorientate oneself for the rest of the day. If the work has been deep and effective, then there may well be thoughts or feelings that you wish to discuss with the practitioner. If feeling deeply relaxed then you will want to take some time to 'wake up' again and get back in touch with your current reality. Many people liken their reaction to some of these treatments as having been in a dream-like state, similar to that experienced just before sleeping.

Both Shiatsu and Jin Shen Do concentrate on working with the individual's own energy, and much will depend on the energetic exchange with the practitioner or therapist. In any form of bodywork, a sense of, and respect for, the individual's energy is most important, although an exchange does also occur in non-contact therapies.

Do-in is a form of shiatsu exercise that you can do for yourself. It is a treatment for the whole body, and is often used as a way of 'waking the body up'. You can use the techniques to work over the whole body in detail, or as a more general tonic. This is different from Shiatsu in being much less specific to individual points or to the meridians, but it is wonderfully invigorating. You can do this every day to generally tone your body and to give an instant energy boost. Consult a Shiatsu practitioner for a more personalized plan.

1. Stand easily, with your knees 'soft' and your feet about hip-width apart. Shake out first your arms, and then your legs, and make this quite energetic. Imagine that you are shaking off the dust of any tension, and letting go of any tightness or stress in your body. Continue to do this for about a minute, loosening up your shoulders, hips, and back as well as your limbs.

2. Now return to your still starting position, and form your hands into loose fists. You are going to use these with very relaxed wrists to gently 'knock' your way along your body. Starting just above your head, let your loose fists fall onto your head from very relaxed wrists. Tap all over the top of your head, letting the weight of your hands do the work. Tap down each side, and down the back of your head, and then down each side of your neck. This should feel stimulating and gently invigorating. It is not meant to hurt at all. Keep the movements relaxed and easy, and you should soon find that you develop a gentle rhythm.

3. Then relax your left hand, and use your right, loosely held fist to knock or tap its way along the top of your left shoulder, and then down your left arm. Take three or four lines

down the length of your arm, tapping all the way down, and then lifting off and returning to the shoulder, until you have worked your way over all your arm. Then use your left, loosely held fist, to work in the same way along your right shoulder, and down your right arm. Remember not to hit yourself, but to keep your wrists relaxed, and let your loosely held fist fall on you, using its weight as the only pressure.

4. Using both hands together now, work your way down your trunk, and down whatever part of your back you can comfortably reach, and then shake out your arms and legs like you did at the start.

5. Next, take a moment or two to work over each buttock, and then use both hands to work down first your left leg, and then your right. Do this as you did with your arms, working down each leg in strips, and returning to the top to work down another strip, until the whole leg has been covered.

6. Balancing carefully, lift first one foot, then the other, and knock your way gently over each sole. Stand for a moment in your relaxed starting position, and take a deep breath.

Your whole body will now have been woken up, and the overall feeling is very uplifting. This releases a lot of energy. The whole exercise can be done in just a few minutes, although you can take longer if you like, or if you experience any areas of your body as being stuck or inflexible. Do this every morning as part of your wake-up routine, or at any point in the day when you feel in need of a pick-me-up.

Finding out more

British School of Shiatsu-Do
188 Old Street
London EC1V 9BP
Tel: 0171 251 0831

Shiatsu Society
14 Oakdene Road
Redhill
Surrey RH1 6BT
Tel: 01737 767896

The Shiatsu Society of Ireland
12 The Cove
Malehide
Co. Dublin
Tel: 01 845 3647

Jin Shen Do Foundation
P.O. Box 1097
Felton, California 95018
U.S.A.
Tel: 408 338 9454

Further Reading

Shizuto Masunaga with Waturu Ohashi, *Zen Shiatsu*, Japan Publications Inc., Tokyo
Miyamoto Musashi, *A Book of Five Rings*, Allison and Busby
Toru Namikoshi, *The Complete Book of Shiatsu Therapy*, Japan Publications Inc., Tokyo.

SKINCARE

Epsom Salt • Salt

The skin is our largest organ of elimination. It plays an important role in our continuing good health, yet we take most of its actions for granted. It is our point of contact with the rest of the world, a protective wrapping, the vehicle of our vital sense of touch, and an important temperature regulator. It contains some three million sweat glands, manufactures vitamin D, denotes racial origin and exposure to the sun, and is a mirror of our health. Weighing some 6–10lb, and covering about two square yards, this remark-ably versatile organ has tremendous powers of elasticity – as witnessed by our ability to grow, put on weight, become pregnant, and even make facial expressions.

We know that our skin is continually renewing itself – losing dead cells and replacing them with new. This is part of the process we witness as cuts and wounds heal. The outer layer of our skin, the epidermis, is composed mainly of dead cells, new ones continuously being made in the inner layer or dermis. We naturally shed thousands of these cells each day, but this cycle, like all other body processes, can become sluggish or in need of support. However good our personal hygiene, there is more we can do to encourage healthy skin function.

The skin shares with the lungs the responsibility for exchanges with the air around us. Your skin breathes too, absorbing oxygen and expelling carbon dioxide formed in the tissues. This explains the great connection between breathing difficulties, like asthma, and skin complaints, like eczema. Looking back through a person's health history, a progression can often be seen from problems in one of these areas to difficulties in another. Long-term smokers often develop dry-skin complaints, and infantile dermatitis, unless properly treated, may disappear only to develop into breathing difficulties as the child grows.

The elimination of uric acid is another skin function (the composition of sweat is very similar to urine). The waste we eliminate from the body in perspiration can take some of the pressure off the kidneys and the liver. The more effective ways there are of ridding waste products from the body, the better it can function. Naturopathy, along with many other healthcare philosophies, maintains that insufficient elimination is a major cause of ill health. Getting rid of what is no longer needed in the body is certainly as necessary as providing it with the right nutrients and building materials.

Simply allowing skin a chance to relax and breathe can be remarkably rejuvenating. A few days off from regular shaving, or wearing make-up shows instant results in a clearer, healthier-looking skin. Air baths are another lovely way of allowing the skin to breathe all over – simply stand near to an open window after a bath or shower, and use your hands to gently massage as much of your body as you can comfortably reach in the stream of fresh air. This gently stimulates all the nerve endings in the skin and results in a glowing feeling all over.

There are enormous benefits to be gained from unclogging the skin by sloughing off the millions of dead cells which can fill the pores. **Dry skin brushing** is one of the most effective ways I know of doing this, and it has other benefits for the body too – stimulating the lymphatic system and pepping up the circulation. Using a natural bristle skin brush, cover the whole body with short or long brushing strokes. Starting on the soles of the feet and working always towards the heart, even the scalp can be brushed in this way. Never brush the face, however, as the skin here is too sensitive. The feeling of an all-over brush is enlivening and invigorating.

Salts in their many guises form a part of any naturopathic repertoire. Ordinary table salt should not, in fact, be on any table, but moved to the bathroom, where it is a wonderful thing. A small handful added to bath water is a useful cleansing agent for women, and is particularly helpful if there is any infection or damaged skin. Larger amounts of salt can be used for a salt rub, or salt glow. This is tremendously stimulating, sloughing off dead skin cells and giving the circulation a boost:

Place 2lb of table salt in a bowl and add enough hot water to form a thick paste. Taking handfuls at a time, rub well over the whole body for a few minutes – rubbing should be vigorous, but not enough to hurt. Shower off with hot water, and then reduce the temperature to finish off with a tepid or cold shower, and towel dry gently. Ideally, follow the salt rub with a short walk or other form of exercise. This is an excellent cleanser, and can be done once a week as part of maintaining a healthy skin and keeping circulation at an optimum. It can also be used locally on areas of dry skin such as feet and elbows: here, though, it is a good idea to follow the salt rub with an application of warmed sesame or olive oil to moisturize it.

Epsom salts also have a role to play. These are pure magnesium, a mineral required for over 80 per cent of all body activities on a cellular level. A hot bath to which 1 lb of epsom salts has been added has a wonderfully cleansing effect on the skin, encouraging perspiration and drawing out impurities. As the magnesium is absorbed, it aids the relaxation of muscles, thereby easing any aches and pains. These baths are deeply relaxing and have an important place in any form of stress management. Ideally, stay in the bath for 20 minutes, then wrap up warmly and either lie down or go to bed. This ensures that the positive effects of the bath will continue and the tiredness becomes a benefit – I often recommend this bath to people who have difficulty relaxing, or trouble in getting to sleep. Epsom salts baths should not be taken if you have eczema, psoriasis or high blood pressure, and women should avoid them during and immediately prior to menstruation as the effects can be depleting at that time. Otherwise, they can be taken up to two times a week.

SPIRITUALITY

Nowadays it seems that we are becoming more open to the idea of a personal connection with the divine. When this knowledge infuses our lives we are able to apply ourselves differently to all manner of challenges, whether they directly concern the health of the body, or the balance and harmony of our whole experience. A strong connection with spirit can often be the missing element in our daily lives. Beyond our material concerns, many people ask themselves at some point in their lives – What am I here for? What is my purpose? or Is there any reason behind or beyond my experiences? Finding the answers to these questions can be one of the most rewarding experiences of our lives.

There is a large number of spiritual ethics that can guide and inform our lives, from being able to trust that our future is safe and does not depend solely on external security, to knowing the sense in not harbouring malicious thoughts, or speaking unkindly about others. Embracing honesty and purity of intent begins with ourselves, and this is a profoundly effective way of enabling ourselves to release addictions and other habit patterns. Once we begin to remember our own place within the world, we can see ourselves in true relationship with others, and we are able to clear our motivations and desires. When we choose to live our lives in harmony then we naturally move towards clear health for our body and our understanding. The world of spirit is our world, and when we accept that we ourselves are spiritual beings, we can begin to find the compassion and care we need to employ for ourselves and for others.

Spirituality and healing are directly linked. We often heal ourselves when we accept that there is more to our lives than the mundane and begin to embrace spiritual values. One of our biggest current spiritual challenges is in learning to accept and embody our physicality. The body is a remarkable thing and a wonderful gift. That we spend so much of our time ignoring it, berating it, and accusing it of letting us down in some way, speaks only of our own ignorance. We need to be able to love ourselves in our current manifestation – the way we are, as a first step towards healing our lives and developing relationships with others. It is very hard to achieve full health when we feel deep down that we do not deserve it, or are not worthy of it, or even that it is not really very important. What a waste of spirit it would be to come here and live the way that we do, in a physical body, if that body were not important to us.

There are marked differences between our established religions, many of which seem to focus on keeping us stuck in negative situations, and the emerging light of the spiritual movement. Individual religions can cause separation, and teach that only those who follow their rules will enter the kingdom of heaven. Such a judgemental position seems at odds with supposed precepts of love and sharing. It is well worth reviewing our beliefs to see whether they are built on guilt and ignorance, or if they can liberate us, light our lives, and lead us forwards. We can ask ourselves if its precepts are alive and relevant to our daily life, and whether is it founded on our own direct experience.

When we feel spiritually nurtured, secure and knowledgeable, we effect a remarkable event – we live our lives at cause. This means we begin to take responsibility for our choices, and realise our birthright. In following the joy that is available to us, we can become co-creators in our own destiny. This means a difference in our health, stress levels, happiness, and also to the way that we live. Our daily habits, mind-set, and what we will accept in our lives can be altered to change our entire experience. Our lives can be a wonderful adventure, and the choice is ours.

If we accept that we are, each one of us, an aspect of the divine, then we have a duty or an obligation to ourselves to be the best that we can be. This can mean being as honourable, ethical, powerful and beautiful as we possibly can, and simply reaching out for the greatness of our potential every minute. It frees us to use tools other than fear, and to recognize the many ways that can lead us to fulfilment. We also have permission to deserve the very best for ourselves in every area of our lives.

Experiencing the spirituality of our own lives is something that we may do at any time, it simply requires us to wake up to it. Consider dedicating your day to your own higher purpose, or

---

taking just a moment with the changing of the light to remember and experience the love that is creation. Stop and see the beauty of a flower, let it register in your heart, or make a commitment to be true to yourself and your beliefs. Choose an issue that is important to you, and do something practical to further its cause.

Take time at the beginning and end of each day to reflect on what has happened, and how at peace you feel with yourself. Review the events of your day, and seek whatever guidance or wisdom you need in order to resolve anything that is outstanding. This enables you to sleep more easily, having cleared your mind, and to begin a new day without carrying too much over into it from previous events.

Remember, too, that this is your life, and you are the most important person in it. Discover what you need to give you peace of mind, an easy conscience, and a clear heart, and act upon it now. This is a true and important quest. Do not let the trivia of the day stand in your way, or the weight of past conditioning. Be true to yourself, and 'walk your talk'.

Allow yourself to relax and become like a child again, secure in the knowledge that your future is safe, and that you have the protection and the guidance that you need. Take care to nurture and care for this childlike you, and do nothing to harm this important aspect of yourself. Recognize the childlike self in others, too, and learn to play!

Further Reading

Neil Freer, *Breaking the God Spell*, Falcon Press
Max Freedom Long, *What Jesus Taught in Secret*, DeVorss Publications
Kenneth Meadows, *Earth Medicine*, Element Books
Jamie Sams and Twylan Nitsch, *Other Council Fires Were Here Before Ours*, Harper.

SUPPLEMENTS

In an ideal world, we would be able to obtain all the nourishment we need from the food we eat. Unfortunately, the growing conditions, shipping, and storage of fresh produce are often geared more towards production targets and ease of transportation rather than to providing and conserving the inherent goodness of the foods themselves. If you are eating food that is grown more than one mile from the sea, has been stored for more than a few hours or has been treated by freezing, drying or canning, then it will have lost some of its nutrient value. We have chemically farmed the land so intensively in recent years, that many of the nutrients that should be present in the soil have disappeared. Iodine, for instance, is only naturally present in soil from areas next to the sea, otherwise it must be added.

An all-round vitamin and mineral supplement, taken on a regular basis will, as its name suggests, supplement your diet and provide you with essential nutrients. They are not alternatives to a well-balanced diet, but will support those efforts and ensure that a full range of nutritional elements is available to the body. These are the essential building blocks for health. They are necessary for growth, repair, and also regulate the metabolism.

The absence or major deficiency of any one vitamin or mineral can endanger the whole body. The mineral calcium, for example, is necessary for the healthy growth of teeth and bones; vitamin A is essential to the health and structure of the skin and eyes; and vitamin C speeds the healing of wounds through its effects on the cells and blood vessels. Vitamins and minerals work together in the body; vitamins A and E need each other to work satisfactorily; iron is important in the prevention of anaemia, but it requires an adequate placing of copper to be effective, and this is regulated by the presence of zinc. Iron uptake may be lowered in the presence of tea, coffee and bran, but vitamin C can greatly aid its absorption. This sometimes complicated synergistic action can be thrown out of balance if one vitamin or mineral is taken in isolation.

While all of us can benefit from a good supply of these materials, certain groups can have greater need of them, or need them more at particular times in their lives. Vitamins and minerals are all essential for growing children; for women during pregnancy and during the menopause, and particularly if taking the contraceptive pill; for the elderly; for athletes or those making special demands on their bodies; and anybody actively destroying vitamins within their body through smoking, drinking or, in some cases, slimming, or experiencing high levels of stress.

A good multi-vitamin and mineral supplement is the best way to ensure a good supply of all these nutrients. It may provide an excess of some substances, but these are usually easily transported out of the body. Individual vitamins or minerals should not be taken on a long-term basis without professional nutritional advice. They all work together in various ways to ensure optimum health. If one particular nutrient is taken in excess, it can throw the whole system out of balance.

The legacy of poor quality food tells in our overall health, and many health professionals will treat individuals with specific vitamins or minerals in isolation to correct particular imbalances or shortcomings in nutritional status. Those of us without specific health problems requiring this sort of treatment will tend to use supplements as an insurance against long-term deficiency, and as a way to maintain optimum health.

You get what you pay for with supplements, and at the cheaper end of the market, additives, synthetic substances and even sugars and saccharine can appear on the list of ingredients. One vitamin C supplement I saw in a high street chain of health food shops contained sugar, orange colouring and orange flavouring all in greater quantities than the vitamin itself. You would have done as well to have just a glass of sugary, vitamin-free orange squash. This makes a nonsense of the whole idea of adding a good, necessary support to your diet. Some supplement suppliers also use synthetic copies rather than the active vitamins and minerals themselves – these behave differently in the body, and can cause confusion at a biochemical level. If one of the reasons for taking supplements is to increase the body's ability to cope – to relieve stresses – then obviously the natural substance will be preferred.

Most naturopaths and nutritional advisors will have investigated the market and will be able to recommend supplements that are of good quality, additive free and hypoallergenic. (This means that the manufacturers will not have used any substances in the packing of the tablets or capsules that are likely to aggravate allergies.) They will also suggest, wherever possible, the actual vitamin, rather than a chemical substitute.

The simple table below shows some of the actions of vitamins and minerals within the body. It is not a good idea to pick just one or two and take those without expert advice. If you can identify an area where you suspect you may be experiencing a deficiency, then the best approach is to pick a broad spectrum supplement which contains a good amount of that substance, or to consult a practitioner. Of course, you could also check that your diet contains adequate amounts of foods that contain it. Vitamins and minerals are usually identified as being present in measurements of milligrams (mg) or micrograms (mcg), although some are measured in international units (IU).

The World Health Organisation has identified minimum daily requirements for many although not all of these micro-nutrients, and these are known as the recommended daily allowance (RDA). Various studies have shown these figures to be the absolute minimum daily allowance; bearing in mind that we will get some vitamins and minerals from the foods we eat (if we are lucky). I suggest these be used as a minimum figure to look for in multi-supplement tablets.

Vitamins:
Vitamin A (retinol) is necessary for the skin and eyes. It is present in oily fish, green vegetables, yellow fruit, carrots and

---

dairy food. The RDA is 2500IU

Vitamin B complex is a range of B Vitamins including folic acid and vitamin B$_{12}$. It is necessary for all tissue growth, the health of the skin, mouth, eyes and hair, function of the nervous system, utilization of protein, liver function, and also works as a blood cleanser, aids fertility and the digestion of carbohydrates. It is found in yeast, wholegrain products, green vegetables, eggs, nuts, some seafood and dairy products, and in meat. The RDA varies as per the individual vitamin.

Vitamin C (ascorbic acid) acts to maintain the health of all cells, blood vessels, gums and teeth, and is vital to wound healing. It can be found in fresh raw vegetables, citrus and other fruits and potatoes. The RDA is 30mg, although much larger doses may be taken to speed healing.

Vitamin D (cholecalciferol) is involved in the formation of teeth and bones, and is necessary to use calcium and phosphorus properly in the body. It can be found in oily fish, butter, eggs and fish liver oils, and the body manufactures it through the effect of sunshine on the skin. The RDA is 200IU

Vitamin E (tocopherol) is essential to fertility, muscle health, and is known as one of the anti-ageing vitamins. It is found in green vegetables, vegetable oils, wheatgerm and nuts. The RDA is 10mg.

Minerals

Calcium is essential to the function of the heart and all enzyme reactions, and is important for the bones, teeth, blood and nerves. It can be found in wholegrains, nuts and seeds, green leafy vegetables and dairy produce. The RDA is 800mg.

Iodine is a component of thyroid hormones controlling growth and metabolism. It is found in seafoods, weeds and vegetables, and all produce that is grown near the sea in iodine-rich soils. The RDA is 200mcg.

Iron is needed for haemoglobin to carry oxygen around the body, and it is also involved in fighting infection. It can be found in whole grains, nuts, green vegetables, molasses, dried apricots and meat. The RDA is 14mg although this will vary enormously, especially during menstruation.

Magnesium is necessary to the growth, repair and maintenance of all cells, and it interacts closely with calcium. It can be found in seafood, nuts, whole grains, dried figs and dates. The RDA is 300mg.

Phosphorus works with calcium for the health of the bones and teeth, and is necessary for the release and use of energy throughout the body. It can be found in milk, cheese, eggs, fish, wheatgerm, nuts and meat. The RDA is 800mg.

Zinc is involved in many hormone actions, and in appetite control and hair growth. It is found in offal, shellfish, fish, green vegetables, cereals, meat and pulses. The RDA is 15mg.

Finding out more
Nutrition Society
10 Cambridge Court
210 Shepherds Bush Road
London W6 7NJ
Tel: 0171 602 0228

Health Plus
Dolphin House
30 Lushington Road, Eastbourne
East Sussex BN21 4LL
Tel: 01323 737374

Lamberts Nutritional Suppliers
1 Lamberts Road
Tunbridge Wells TN2 3EQ
Tel: 01892 513116

FSC Supplements
The Health and Diet Food Co. Ltd.
Europa Park, Stoneclough Road
Radcliffe, Manchester M26 1GG
Tel: 01204 707420

Sona Nutritional Suppliers
IDA Business Centre, IDA Industrial Park
Whiteheaven, Dublin 24
Tel: (353) 1 4515087

Incorporated Society of British Naturopaths
Kingston
The Coach House, 293 Gilmerton Road
Edinburgh EH16 5UQ
Tel: 0131 664 3435

Further Reading

Dr Stephen Davies and Dr Alan Stewart, *Nutritional Medicine*, Pan Books
Earl Mindell, *The Vitamin Bible*, Arlington Books
Ross Trattler ND DO, *Better Health through Natural Healing*, Thorsons.

TALKING THERAPIES

Analytic • Cognitive • Behavioural • Humanistic • Transference

There are many branches of psychotherapy, all with their own specific techniques, approaches and philosophies. All deal with psychological, emotional and practical difficulties through a variety of talking skills. Sometimes this involves discussing what is happening both in the client's life and in the relationship with the therapist, and having the benefit of the therapist's insights and interpretation. Other times, specific skills and techniques may be used to facilitate understanding and change. Common to all these approaches is a desire to help the client manage their lives more effectively, and complete confidentiality.

Throughout our lives we are continually assessing and/or reaching to our effectiveness and our own happiness and contentment. The degree to which we can be successful in our own scheme of things is reliant on a number of different factors. The way that we understand the world to be, and our own position in it, colours our actions and expectations as fully as do opportunity and ability. In much the same way as an old injury can be a recurring physical difficulty, so an old emotional hurt can cause difficulties responding to things appropriately today. Psychotherapy can offer a way of reaching back to the cause of any discomfort in a safe, supported way, and allow healing and understanding.

It is the skills of the therapist and the sense of containment and support offered by the commitment to working in this way that marks the psychotherapies as distinct. Many people choose this as an aid to personal growth, to foster their own sense of individual responsibility, and as a way of effecting and managing change in their lives. When we work to refine the physical level of our existence, an understanding of our own emotional and psychological well-being is intrinsic to our overall view of things.

Most therapists will work with a client on either a short-term contract basis, which is useful for working with specific issues, and to allow the establishment of a trusting relationship or as an ongoing process. An initial commitment is usually required to a mutually agreed number of appointments, although this may be as few as two or three. Some therapists do not charge for their consultation or initial appointment because this is the time when they and the client are interviewing each other, and determining whether a commitment to working together would be appropriate. During this initial meeting, the therapist should be able to explain just how they work, and what you might expect from the sessions. It is useful at this stage if you can be as frank and clear about your own situation and expectations.

This is also the time when matters that are important to you may be raised – questions about the therapist's training and experience, and any matters of political awareness, sexual orientation, or knowledge of a particular area of life that you feel will make a difference.

The relationship with a therapist can be such an important one that it is vital to feel that they can be warm, caring, honest and understanding. This initial interview will be a time when you need to make an initial assessment as to these qualities, and whether an ongoing therapeutic relationship with this therapist would be beneficial. You may arrive at therapy during a time of crisis, and be looking to receive valuable support, a route to understanding your current situation in terms of why it has occurred, how to survive it, and a way to make plans for the future. The therapist's role is not to rescue you, but to help find ways for you to work with the fabric of your life to weave a better way.

Psychotherapy falls into four main branches: analytic, humanistic, cognitive and behavioural. In practice, many therapists use a combination of different approaches, and some work solely with the client's own ideas and experiences, while others add their own insights, understandings and interventions.

Analytic psychotherapy is based on the findings of Freud and later Jung (see Self Analysis, pp. 261–7). It concentrates on the links between our different levels of awareness and the interplay between our conscious understanding, and the workings of the unconscious.

Cognitive psychology maintains that the way we understand the world now is based on the views and assumptions that were generated by personal experiences. By exploring new possibilities and adopting other points of view, we can change our behaviour.

The **behavioural approach** places great emphasis on our environment. Some of our actions receive rewards, e.g. they make us feel good, while other behaviours attract some form of punishment or deprivation. Recognition of these facts and learning more 'good' behaviours can lead to more appropriate ways of behaving.

Humanistic psychotherapy seeks to uncover and work with each individual's own unique experience, affirming their own personal view of the world, and strengthening their ability to act from their own truth.

All of these approaches recognize the importance of the mind–body link to varying degrees, and many therapists will place great emphasis on the physical sensations, postures and communications of their client. Although working mainly in the emotional or psychological arena, psychotherapy recognizes the role of feelings in health problems, and that on occasion they can be a cause of physical symptoms.

Depending on the therapist's training, sessions may involve clients enacting old conflicts and finding new resolutions to them; applying a new understanding to established patterns of behaviour, and learning to recognize how habitual responses can colour current attitudes and relationships. Much of this work is uncovered through talking, and the structure that is imposed upon this will lead to some form of resolution. Other techniques, like psychodrama, dream analysis, creative exercises, movement and visualizations may also be used. 'Homework' may be suggested in the form of exercises or pursuits that the client may wish to do in order to further their progress between sessions. Ideally, the benefit and insights from individual sessions will make a difference to daily life, and become part of a new way of coping.

Perhaps one of the best known therapeutic techniques is 'chair' or 'parts' work. This involves inviting an imaginary visitor to the session to sit in and become involved in the process that is being worked on. This might be a parent, colleague, friend or anybody the client feels the need to address. It may also be a part of themselves. This affords the opportunity to experiment with addressing the person, hearing what they might have to say, seeing how it feels to be near them, etc. This can be a very useful technique if trying to resolve issues from the past when it would be inappropriate, or not possible, to approach the person directly. It is also a good way to experience and express uncomfortable feelings like anger and vulnerability, while in the safety of the therapy room. After talking to whoever is in the 'chair', the client may choose to sit there themselves, and see how it feels and whether they have any response. This technique can be used to isolate different parts of the self, like the inner critic, or ringleader, or witness, and allow some useful dialogue. It is also a good way to identify different parts of the self, and gives the chance to experience what it is like without different personality parts.

This type of work forms a major part of Gestalt therapy, which takes place both in individual sessions and in groups. Other forms of therapy may also be extended into a group situation and many therapists run such groups alongside their work with individuals. A common set-up is for the therapist to invite someone into their group after working with them individually for a while. This may mark an end to the individual sessions, or may be an additional support to ongoing work. The group members are usually all dealing with a particular issue or area of their lives, and sharing the experience with others can be very beneficial.

Among the many other forms of therapy are trans-personal, personal construct, existential, process-oriented, feminist and transference-based. **Transference** is an analytic term for the feelings that are projected onto others, and in this case, onto the therapist. Sometimes these can form a stong unconscious bond between people, and maybe feelings that the client finds too uncomfortable to own for themselves. An awareness of them, through open discussion, can be both a liberating and transforming experience.

Many therapists work individually, either in their own homes or in clinics. Sometimes a group of therapists may form a group practice. Individual appointments last between fifty minutes and one hour, and double sessions may sometimes be booked. It is common to see a therapist once a week, although twice weekly or more is not unusual, varying between therapists, and according to how the process is developing.

Therapist training involves many hours of individual and group therapy for them, as well as the theoretical content of their course. Most practitioners continue their own therapy while they are in practice, and they can also receive supervision on their case-load from another thera-pist. Some schools encourage therapists to see clients before they have completed their training, and this work is always carefully supervised by a trainer or lecturer. When working in this way, the client will always be informed, and a lower fee is charged. The fees for psychotherapy vary enormously between practitioners. Usually, the more experienced therapists will charge more, but a high fee is no guarantee of a better practitioner – there are many other factors to take into account such as the costs of running their practice. Many therapists have a sliding scale of fees, so those on low incomes can receive some concession.

Finding out more
Association of Group and Individual Psychotherapists
1 Fairbridge Road
London N19 3EW
Tel: 0171 272 7013
Association for Humanistic Psychology
26 Huddlestone Road
London E7 0AN
Tel: 0181 555 3077
British Association of Psychotherapists
37 Mapesbury Road
London NW2
Tel: 0181 452 9823

Further Reading

D. Brown and J. Pedder, *Introduction to Psychotherapy*, Routledge & Kegan Paul
Irene Claremont de Castillejo, *Knowing Woman*, Harper & Row
Jay Haley, *Uncommon Therapy*, Norton.

VISUALIZATIONS

The use of the imagination to create pictures in the mind of a desired situation or condition is not new. Informally we can call this daydreaming, but when we structure and focus this work it can become a powerful tool. Our imagination is one of our most valuable and useful assets, and harnessing its tremendous power can prove to be a truly transformational experience. Using our imagination can let us daydream, help us survive difficult experiences and provide innovative solutions to problems and challenges. Consciously working with the imagination provides us with a clear link to our dreams and desires.

There are different visualization techniques, but in general the more powerfully and completely you can picture your desired image, the greater its effectiveness. You can visualize your desires for a few minutes each day, thereby renewing your vision and keeping it as a priority in your life. This can be done at a regular time, or in conjunction with other techniques for achieving change, like using affirmations (see pp. 14–17). You can visualize anything that your imagination will stretch to, and the real purpose of this technique is to centre your attention on a desired goal or change that you are actively working towards – you have to take action as well as daydream, however well-structured it is.

The object of your desire can be anything from a career change – where you can picture the new job, work environment, colleagues, what you will wear, the journey to and from home, etc. – to inner changes in psychological response, emotional patterns or more physical health concerns.

When starting to work with your imagination in this way, it is a good idea to begin with something fairly simple, and it is always advisable to choose something that is well within your sphere of influence. Developing your imagination and your will is just like developing a muscle; it helps to start in a relatively small way, and then build on those early successes. The body responds wonderfully well to being united in its purpose with the mind in this way. Visualizations are often used to effect changes in everything from shape to immune status. An important part of every exercise in weight training and body building is imaging the effect on the muscle or muscle group that is being worked. Seeing the increase in muscle size and the increased definition of the area in your mind sets up a powerful and immediate connection between mind and body, ensuring that every resource is focused on the job in hand. Studies have shown that performing these exercises without this mental participation does not result in such good progress.

Our bodies respond fully to our ideas and beliefs of how they should be. When we feel happy we tend to move more freely and easily, without conscious thought. When we smile and laugh a whole range of beneficial physiological changes are set in motion, improving everything from our ability to continue feeling good, to our rate of digestion. Visualizing ourselves to be in warm, nurturing situations has the same effect as actually being there. This is a common form of visualization – taking an imaginary journey to a place of beauty where we can be renewed, and explore the beneficial feelings and sensations that engenders. For some this place might be a lush green valley or a sun-drenched beach. The detail, and the layers of depth and colour that you can build into your visualization are part of what will make it successful.

You can buy relaxation tapes, and these often include some form of visualized journey, or guided imagery – these are the same thing only the ideas and suggestions as to where you are and what you might be experiencing are provided for you. Another beneficial use of visualizations is to imagine the state of your body and its inner functions. Current research is proving the remarkable effects of these techniques on lowering blood pressure, improving immune status and speeding recovery from illness. Focusing on recovery from a cold, for instance, by visualizing the mucous membranes slowly drying, and the lymphatic system quickly disposing of waste materials while all your muscles relax, really can make a difference.

The key is to make the visualization work for you. If you want to stimulate your immune system, or elevate your antibody activity, choose an image that will be meaningful for you. People often suggest you see your body's defences rather like an army on the march, but this might be a rather difficult image for the peacemakers amongst us. Seeing it as a baseball team or a football team may work better for sports fans, or a sea of Pacman images for computer games buffs, or as colourful abstract images for those who are artistically inclined or design based.

When visualizations are used in conjunction with another technique for achieving success, like affirmations, the results can be remarkable. One of the best ways to combine these two powerful aids is to spend some time visualizing your desire each day, and then to develop an affirmation to support this. Repeating the affirmation at times during the day continues the work of the earlier imagining, and repeating the visualization process again at the end of the day completes the process.

If you want something to happen, it makes every sense to concentrate, and to use every possible aid in order to achieve it. Unlocking the powers of imagination yields tremendous benefits as it overflows into other areas of your life and re-establishes the connections between what you think, who you are, and what you do.

Successful visualizations

- be sure about what you want to happen
- make as clear a picture as you can
- include detail, shading, and depth to make as real an image as possible
- use images that have strong meanings for you, and make the visualization as relevant as you can
- spend time developing your visualization to make it as useful as possible
- attach as much energy as possible to your visualization by spending time on it at least twice a day

---

- reinforce your visualizations with techniques like affirmations
- be prepared to experience the change you are working for.

Beyond using visualizations to image desired events or outcomes of situations, use this technique called **structural tension**. This is a lovely development that acknowledges where we are now, as well as where we want to be, and uses the fact that there is a difference between those two places to generate more energy for change. It is a simple technique that can have very dramatic effects.

Make a clear mental picture of your desire, with as much detail and colour as possible, then find a picture that will sum up your current reality or situation, and make that as clear as you can. Take some time to fill out both images. Now, spend a few minutes seeing the picture of your current reality, and then switch to seeing yourself living your dream. Give enough time to each image to allow yourself to really feel what it is like, and then move on to the other one. To-ing and fro-ing between the separate reality sets causes a sort of tension, linking the two and then working to draw them closer together.

Further Reading

Richard Nelson Bolles, *What Colour is Your Parachute*, Ballantine Books
Kenneth Meadows, *The Medicine Way*, Element Books
Barbara Sher with Annie Gottlieb, *Wishcraft*, Ballantine Books.

WOMEN'S HEALTHCARE

This is an area where natural therapies and techniques can be particularly beneficial. There are some good hydrotherapy (pp. 141–2) measures for enhancing vaginal health, and the acidity of the body, which is determined to a large part by diet, can directly influence the incidence of disturbance in this area. (The pH or acidity of the vagina is inversely proportional to the pH of the rest of the body – when the body is slightly alkaline, as it should be, the vagina becomes slightly acidic. This makes it an unwelcome place for thrush and other invading organisms.)

The problems of painful, absent or heavy periods respond well to herbal (p. 129) and naturopathic treatments; their gentle effects encouraging the body to find its own natural balance. Menstruation has a negative image for some people, and the combination of positive supportive measures and counselling can reinforce the beneficial potential of this special time. The monthly cycle also provides a good sense of timing on which detoxification programmes (p. 85) and health regimens can be based.

Natural contraception and fertility control are among a range of self-care approaches. This method of pinpointing the fertile time in each cycle can help relieve couples of the burden of full-time contraception, or, indeed, aid them in their attempts to conceive. Every month, at the time of ovulation when the woman becomes fertile, there are changes in both her basal or resting temperature and the mucous secretions of her vagina. These can both be measured quite easily. The basal temperature can be taken immediately on waking each morning, and the vaginal secretions tested for viscosity or stickiness. Noted over a couple of months, it is soon easy to see at what point ovulation occurs, even for those with irregular cycles. The only difficulty with this method is that sex can interfere with it! The presence of secretions, creams, etc. in the vagina can upset the mucous reading, and the excitement of a relationship can alter the basal temperature. If this is the case, the findings may need to be charted over a longer period of time to enable a clear pattern to emerge. Nowadays, this natural method may be less than useful as a means of contraception because of the need for protection from disease which only the barrier methods and safer sex practices can provide.

A number of women record the changes in their cycle even though they are not sexually active. Should a relationship develop, they then have a strong record to refer to, but perhaps more important is the feeling of knowing one's own body a little better. Regular breast checks and even gynaecological self-examination are further examples of this wise concern over how our bodies function. It is a good idea for a woman to examine her breasts each month, ideally just after a period or on a fixed date; this is advisable from the point of view of recognizing any changes in breast appearance and texture, but also in reuniting us with this area.

Unless breast-feeding or in a sexual relationship, it is very easy not to pay any attention at all to our 'sexual' areas, and I feel this diminishes us. Well-illustrated leaflets on breast examination can still be found at most health clinics and well-woman centres. Speculums for gynaecological self-examination can be bought at any chemist, and again a range of clinics can advise on their use for those who have never been examined with one. A mirror and some photos of healthy vaginas and cervixes are all that is needed. This is not a substitute for regular pap or smear tests.

Natural childbirth is a rapidly growing choice for women in the West. Deciding to allow the body's own pain-killers to do their work is an obvious choice for a healthy woman – pharmaceuticals and surgical intervention have their place for use in emergencies. I am not advocating painful delivery, but more and more women are discovering that if they are relaxed and have support during labour, and have prepared themselves by learning breathing and focusing techniques, then such interventions *may* not be needed. There are many birthing classes around the country which include pre-natal exercises to help stretch the ligaments and improve muscle tone; it is often easier to get back into shape after delivery if you remain active during pregnancy, and these can also help to make the birth easier. Another important factor is the choice of location – some women feel more relaxed at the prospect of a home delivery, while others prefer the reassurance of a hospital birth.

Although it is important to consider the potential risks, as well as the benefits, when deciding where to have a baby, women should always have the choice – in many areas the medical profession tries to make it difficult for women who choose a home delivery. Not only then must the decision be made as early as possible, but it may also be necessary to employ an independent midwife if a home birth is wanted. The National Childbirth Trust is a wonderful resource for more detailed information, and their counsellors can also help with any breast-feeding queries and information on baby allergies (one of the most common allergies in babies is to cow's milk!). There are a number of herbs which can be taken as teas during the later stages of pregnancy to help delivery. Individual assessment is necessary to ensure their safety and efficacy, but both raspberry leaf and lady's mantle can be taken once a day when the birth day is due. A cup of either sort of tea, sipped slowly while it is still warm, can help relax the abdominal muscles and reduce tension.

Many women find that hydrotherapy can also be useful both during and after the birth – warm, moist, towels placed over the diaphragm in the early stages of labour can help relieve the pain of contractions; and massage of the abdomen, shoulders and lower back can be a comfort. It is well worth consulting a naturopath or a well-woman centre if a home birth is desired, as they should be able to make the right suggestions to help make the time as easy and joyous as possible.

Breast examination

Choose a time a few days after menstruation, or if you do not have periods, then pick a regular date every month. Set aside 15–20 minutes to do this for the first few monthly examinations, after that they can be completed in about five minutes.

1. Begin by looking at your breasts when standing in front of a mirror. Note their asymmetry, their contour, the positioning of your nipples and their overall appearance. Look at both side views, and then lean forwards towards the mirror, and again observe the general outline of your breasts as they fall away from your chest wall. Initially, this will be a process of familiarizing yourself with the general appearance of your breasts, any unusual puckering or changes in fullness will then be more easily apparent.

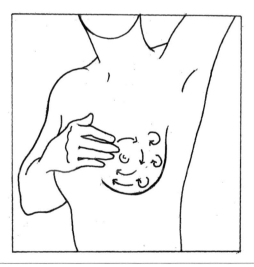

2. Next, lie down on your back and bend one arm, placing the hand underneath your head. This allows full access to the breast and armpit for your other hand. Using the flat of your fingers held together, make small circular pressing movements on the outermost border of your breast. Work your way around the outside of your breast, including an investigation of your armpit, until a full circle is completed. Continue covering your breast in this way, making smaller and smaller circles until you reach your nipple. Notice the colour and appearance of your nipple and its hardness, then repeat the procedure on your other breast.

Most breasts feel glandular, or bumpy, when examined in this way, and with practice you will soon be able to differentiate between what is normal for you and any changes in texture or feel.

Finding out more
Foresight
28 The Paddock
Godalming
Surrey GU7 1XD
Irish Childbirth Trust
17 Dame Court
Dublin 2
Tel: 01 679 4055
National Childbirth Trust
Alexandra House
Oldham Terrace
London W3 6NH
Tel: 0171 992 8637

Women's Health Information Centre
52 Featherstone Street
London EC1Y 8RT
Tel: 0171 251 6580
Terrance Higgins Trust
52–54 Gray's Inn Road
London WC1X 8SO
Tel: 0171 242 1010

Further Reading

Mamatoto, A Celebration of Birth, The Body Shop, Virago
Irene Claremont de Castillejo, *Knowing Woman*, Harper and Row
Angela Phillips and Jill Rakusen, *Our Bodies, Ourselves*, Penguin
Penelope Shuttle and Peter Redgrove, *The Wise Wound*, Palladin
Belinda Grant Viagas, *Natural Healthcare for Women*, Newleaf.

XYZ...

This book contains a reservoir of health-giving alternatives for those with any specific complaint, and it can be dipped into for a wealth of ideas on lifestyle change and the promotion of full health.

There are many more natural therapies developing all the time, and whenever a committed practitioner aligns their skills and their intuition, their own style of work is born. Some natural therapies, like the Bates method of eyesight care, have not been covered here, and also omitted is the heat-sensing Kirlian photography that is used by some practitioners to aid diagnosis. When considering exploring a branch of healthcare, ask yourself whether it is a natural way – one that will support and encourage your own journey towards full health, and honour your own unique prescription of constitutional strengths and challenges.

An important aspect of natural healthcare is its role in ongoing health education. Although most people arrive at a consultation with specific health concerns, a growing number of people now come while in good health, wanting advice on improving their constitution, ensuring continuing optimum health, or information on how to encourage full health in their children. This points to a new way for people to take power and control in their own lives and manage their own health and well-being.

Through information we gain the freedom to make choices, and informed choice is fundamental to sovereignty over our own bodies, our own lives. Reflexologists may access the unified organism through the feet, aromatherapists via the nose – in many cases the choice rests with you.

Other useful addresses
The Bates Association
Friars Court, 11 Tarmount Lane
Shoreham-by-Sea
West Sussex BN43 6RQ
The Breakthrough Centre
7 Poplar Mews, Uxbridge Road
London W12 7JS
Tel: 0181 749 8525
Council for Complementary and Alternative Medicine
Suite D, Park House,
206–208 Latimer Road
London W10 6RE
Tel: 0181 968 3862
Irish Association of Holistic Medicine
9–11 Grafton Street
Dublin 2
Tel: 01 671 2788
What Drs. Don't Tell You
4 Wallace Road
London N1 2PG

Compassion in World Farming
20 Lavant Street
Petersfield
Hants GU32 3EW
Movement for Compassionate Living
47 Highlands Road
Leatherhead
Surrey KT22 8NQ
Institute for Complementary Medicine
15 Tavern Quay
London SE16 1QZ
Tel: 0171 237 5165
Permanent Publications
Hyden House Ltd
Little Hyden Lane
Clanfield
Hampshire PO8 0RU
Tel: 01705 569500

To contact the author for details of workshops and training and for information about her postal advice service, write to:
Belinda Grant Viagas
PO Box 13386
London NW3 2ZE